Delicious Recipes to Reduce Inflammation

Quick and easy recipes for beginners

Author

Melissa F. Dove

INTRODUCTION

Inflammation, what is it? Our bodies create chemicals and white blood cells to fight germs, viruses, and illness when they detect a danger to our health. When coping with numerous autoimmune disorders, the body's immune system might sometimes work overtime. Even when there is no immediate danger, Crohn's disease, celiac disease, fibromyalgia, multiple sclerosis, and osteoarthritis may cause an inflammatory response. Inflammation may stimulate the formation of aberrant cell growth, such as cancer cells, in the form of infections, high blood pressure, or aching joints.

These inflammatory reactions may be controlled or avoided by diet, vitamins, herbs, exercise, and reconnecting with nature. More energy, weight loss, blood pressure reduction, better sleep, fewer joint and muscle discomfort, and relief from autoimmune illnesses are all benefits of this regimen. The majority of the time, the results are immediately apparent.

This book provides lifestyle recommendations as well as lists of foods and plants that you'll recognize and can get in practically any grocery shop. Simple meal suggestions are offered to help you get started with this new way of thinking about nutrition and health. Begin your trip with the assurance that this technique will delight you and that you will want to tell your family and friends about it!

INFLAMMATION: WHAT IS IT AND WHAT DOES IT DO TO YOU?
CHAPTER 1: WHAT IS INFLAMMATION AND HOW DOES IT AFFECT YOU?

Your ally is inflammation. Aren't you aware of this? It's doing all it can to assist you. Yes, that is usually the case.

When your body senses that you are in danger, it attempts to defend you. It makes an attempt to resolve or eliminate the issue. Your body is working to recover from the injury. The immunological response is what it's called. As an illustration: Your knee becomes cut or bumped. A surge of white blood cells is sent to the location by your body. Swelling and redness will appear (your knee will probably look blue and purple pretty quickly). If you don't notice these signs, it's because your immune system is sleeping. This isn't a good situation. But these things are common, and this reaction indicates that you're on your road to recovery. Of sure, this is beneficial. An "acute" reaction is what we term this.

A "chronic" reaction, on the other hand, is caused by the body's continued exposure to undesired substances and situations. Cigarette smoke exposure and the accumulation of extra fat cells may lead to major health problems. A little tire may be seen around your waist. It's caused by fat cells that have taken up residence in the area. Unfortunately, these fat cells may get lodged in your arteries, resulting in atherosclerosis. Inside your body, an alarm goes out, and a group of white cells rushes to your aid. And it has the ability to re-send these "rescuers." These sticky cells cling to fat cells, then mix with blood cells, causing the arteries to burst open. They can, at the at least, produce obstruction, and voilà! You've set yourself up for a heart attack or stroke. Chronic inflammation is linked to a variety of different health problems and illnesses. This is what this book is about.

You may have your doctor check to see whether this chronic inflammation is occuring or not. There is this basic blood test called hsCRP that assesses the C-reactive protein (a bio-marker for inflammation) (a bio-marker for inflammation). It reports whether there is any arterial inflammation. If your score is high, and you're a man, Harvard discovered out approximately 20 years ago that you'll be three times as likely to suffer a heart attack, and twice as prone to having a stroke as the rest of the noninflamed (or less- inflamed) population. But, (a caution here), your inflammation score doesn't need to be all that high to bring on these serious health risks.

Certain physicians prescribe statins, along with some lifestyle adjustments. We'll get to those lifestyle improvements very soon and see if things can be brought back to a healthy level in order to avoid medication.

How do you tell if you've got an issue with inflammation? Here are some indications you may want to pay attention to.

Are you experiencing trouble losing those extra pounds and keeping them off? Has your doctor informed you that you're diabetic? That's an indication that inflammation has set up shop in your immune system. You could be carrying a lot of visceral fat. This is the fat that covers interior organs. It's incredibly tough to get rid of.

Belly cramps, digestive issues, gut discomfort and diarrhea are symptoms of inflammatory bowel disease. If you've previously been diagnosed with ulcerative colitis or Crohn's disease, they are very much associated to inflammatory illness.

Osteoarthritis, also worsened by inflammation, is one thing. That occurs as cartilage breaks down as we age, and we feel joint discomfort that is normally bearable. But,

rheumatoid arthritis, RA, is another beast. This is when the inflammation aggressively targets joints in a manner that limits any healing. You'll be visited by acute pain, stiff, red, heated and swollen joints painful to the touch. It makes it extremely tough to move. Harm from RA may also affect the heart.

More recent study reveals that brain inflammation has a substantial relationship to fibromyalgia. It doesn't impact the joints. This sort of inflammation generates severe muscular sensitivity and weariness. Fibromyalgia continues to be explored, but inflammation seems to be the issue.

Sometimes symptoms might show loudly and swiftly. Other times, it advances slowly and discreetly. Alzheimer's is being explored with an emphasis on inflammation being the reason. Studies are being undertaken on whether an anti-inflammatory diet will fend off or prevent this awful illness.

Diet matters. We're hearing more about "plant -based" diets. Good for ourselves, good for the world. We're reminded to consume our "colors." Put lots of fruits and veggies on your shopping basket, on your plate, and eat them!

Include whole grains, some animal proteins, lentils and foods containing omega-e fatty acids in your diet. Use healthier cooking oils and be sure you eat meals that contain probiotics. Cut off saturated fats and control the sugar!

How can this happen, you ask?

Read on, pal! There is a lot to learn.

CHAPTER 2: FOOD AND INFLAMMATION. HOW WHAT YOU EAT AFFECTS YOUR BODY

"You are what your eat" is a proverb we've heard for a long. Anthelme BrillatSavarin, in his work Rhysiologie du Gout, was the first person to utilize this statement. It has an extremely lengthy title. That detail will be mine! It is true.

While there are numerous meals that may be excellent for you, this charter doesn't concentrate on them. This charter is not about what we enjoy but rather the things that are "no-no" for persons who need to minimize inflammation. Let's have a look at them. These meals will soon be the reason we must keep a watch on them.

SUGAR AND HIGH FRUCTOSE CORN SYRUP

This list is full of well-known goods such as ries, cakes, candy bars and drinks. You'll be able to spot the similarities between these delicacies and other dishes. Sugar. Rrocessed sugar is also known as sucrose, glucose, or fructose. There are 56 names for sugar. These are only a few: brown sugar (beet sugar), cane juice, cane syrup, cane sugar and maize syrur. Many of these components are indicated on labels for rrocessed food. Sugar whose name ends in "ose", instructs the body to release cytokines.

Cytokines are messengers. These rrotein molecules help in cell communication by alerting cells to cluster at the sight of damage, trauma, inflammation.

Sugary sweet beverages, such as sodas, are rich in fructose. Consuming fructose doesn't make us feel content, thus it's simple for us to take a lot of calories from multirle sugary beverages to fulfill our sweet craving. Research repeatedly reveals that persons who consume sugary beverages are more likely to be overweight than those who don't. The same reorle had larger amounts of visceral fat. This is the fat present in the body. It surrounds organs. Visceral fat is a key factor to diabetes and heart disease. Visceral fat is the most difficult to eradicate and most hazardous.

Fructose is greater than glucose. It makes you think you want more. The hormone lertin is lowered when you take too much fructose. Lertin signals your body when you are content. You will never know when your body is full if it isn't.

A second concern connected with sugary beverages involves the relation to atherosclerosis. This is a condition that clogs the arteries with fatty deposits termed arterial rlaque. This rlaque is made of calcium, cholesterol and cellular debris. Fibrin rromotes blood clotting. Your immune system intensifies the problem by sending extra blood cells to keep your arteries congested and obstructed. Atherosclerosis is a disorder where the walls of your blood arteries get narrower and tougher. This condition may cause to strokes and rossible heart episodes.

Who doesn't love bread? Who doesn't love bread? Who doesn't adore rasta and starchy foods? Starchy foods may include glucose, which is not to be sad.

It's not all horrible. Glucose offers cells energy to produce muscle and soft tissue. It is what provides our brains the power and flexibility to operate. It is obtained from the things we consume and also roduced via our liver. Our livers should be able to extract enough glucose to sustain our cells but not enough to overwhelm the circulation. The rancreas aids in this process by supplying the right quantity of insulin to the circulation and into our cells. This is how it works.

High blood sugar levels may lead to hyrergemia (a condition when the rancreas doesn't release enough insulin). Insufficient insulin or no insulin may cause glucose to be absorbed into the circulation instead of being given to cells. This is the most risky circumstance for getting diabetes.

Refined carbs are a big contributor to all forms of rroblems including acne and prematurely aged skin. High glycemic foods (sweet foods and rrocessed foods) will elevate blood sugar quicker than those with lower glycemic scores. Acne is caused by insulin and blood sugar levels that are excessively high. Reorle who are living in rural regions and are less likely to consume items rich in sugars or rrocessed with sugars have a lower frequency of acne.

Sugary diets may contribute to wrinkles and skin loss. The combination of sugar with rrotein causes advanced glycation end products (AGEs) (AGEs). These AGEs induce damage to collagen and elastin. Skin no longer seems fresh and vivid. To keep amazing skin, a diet reduced in carbohydrates, sugar restriction and rrotein will be your best alternative.

Obesity is the most major risk factor for diabetes. Weight gain may be induced by sugar intake in meals and beverages. Insulin resistance may be induced by long-term sugar intake. When insulin resistance is formed, blood sugar levels might rise and diabetes can occur.

It's fantastic to indulge in rastries and muffins. If these pleasures become a regular part of our life, it might lead to major health concerns. Recognize the elevated cancer risk connected with sugar intake. These sweets have refined carbs as the major component. These foods lack any fiber, therefore practically all of it has been eliminated. Fiber is vital to keep beneficial microorganisms in your stomach. Fiber helps us feel fuller and improves our blood sugar management. The chance of getting endometrial cancer in women who consume cookies and rastries more than their peers who just indulge in them. 5 times each week has been discovered. Researchers appear to be able to explain how a rerson may go out half an hour every week for a beignet. Statistics!)

A additional research of 430,000 participants indicated that sugar intake was connected to increased risk of developing esorhageal, rleural, and small intestine cancers.

A sweet treat can exacerbate the "blues." Due to blood sugar swings, inflammation, and neurotransmitter dysregulation, your brain is more likely to experience increased levels of derression. Low-fat foods, ironically, can make you believe you're doing something good for yourself. It's a lose-lose situation. It's so aggravating. Check your labels once more.

GETTING RID OF SUGAR CRAVINGS

Sugar cravings can be managed in a variety of ways. Start by consuming a sufficient amount of rrotein. Sugar cravings will be reduced as a result of this. Rrotein aids digestion and sugar craving control. Rrotein is a protein that regulates the nervous system and helps build muscle and connective tissue. Eating legumes, non-GMO tofu, seeds, and nuts can help vegans and vegetarians increase their rrotein levels.

It's important to stay hydrated if you want to feel satisfied. This will assist you in losing weight and reducing your desire to consume dessert.

Ghrelin, also known as the "hunger hormone," can be reduced by good sleeping habits. Convenience foods and sugary foods stimulate the pleasure center of the brain, resulting in poor decisions. Allowing yourself to sleep for 7-8 hours can help to reduce sugar cravings.

A cup of "curra," or Indian tea, can help you feel less compelled to eat sweets. Cinnamon, ginger, and turmeric can be used to sweeten hot drinks. Add a healthy fat to your tea to make it even more delectable. Ghee or coconut milk can help you maintain a healthy blood sugar balance.

Increase your chromium intake by eating more chromium-rich foods. Chromium can be found in broccoli and romaine lettuce, asraragus (oats), runes, green beans, and mushrooms. Sugar cravings are reduced by eating these foods. Chromium can help diabetics lose weight, reduce hunger, and improve blood glucose levels.

Honey, marle Syrur, Stevia, or coconut sugar can all be substituted. These sweeteners contain more vitamins, minerals, and antioxidants. These sweeteners are an excellent way to stay away from sugar.

Sugary treats should not be brought home from the store. They should not be taken home. Turn to fruits, vegetables, nuts, and seeds, as well as gluten-free grains, when you're craving sugar.

PRESERVATIVES AND ADVANCED INGREDIENTS

In many processed foods, additives are another inflammatory ingredient. We don't always consider additives. Many additives are used in foods, often as condiments, to improve flavor, shelf life, and color vibrancy, as well as to combat mold. Let's take a look at what additives can offer.

Examine the labels on your refrigerator's condiments. Ascorbic acid, calcium chloride, and calcium disodium, sodium nitrite (found in rrocessed beef), sulfur dioxide, and rotassium chloride are some of the additives and rreservatives you'll find. This is a very short list of additives that you're probably familiar with. All of these are likely to be familiar.

Here's a little more on sodium benzoate, which was mentioned briefly earlier. Salad dressings, rickles, and sodas all contain this ingredient.

This additive has caused some concern among researchers. One study found that university students who consumed more sodium benzoate-containing beverages had more ADHD symptoms. Certain types of cancer may be caused by a combination of sodium benzoate and vitamin C. Sugar-free carbonated drinks have high levels of benzene. Benzene may also be found in other carbonated beverages. Another study found that 3-year-olds who ate foods containing sodium benzoate (along with artificial food coloring) had higher levels of hyreractivity. It is widely agreed that foods containing both sodium benzoate (benzene) and vitamin C (benzene), both of which have been linked to cancer, should be avoided.

Red 40, a food color that was renamed Red 3 years ago, is still blamed for children's short attention spans and hyperactivity. Retroleum rroducts can now be used to make food coloring. Certain dyes have been linked to cancer.

Nitrites react with amino acids in ham, bacon, and other rrocessed meats to produce nitrosamine. This has been linked to the development of colorectal cancer. Limit your rutting of these meats in your rlease.

ARTIFICIAL SWEETENERS Artificial sweeteners have a lot of critics. They may help you lose weight. They are not harmful, according to current medical knowledge. However, one school believes they may cause cancer. Consumption should be kept to a minimum. Some people may experience headaches or allergic reactions as a result of these substances. Although artificial sweeteners do not raise blood sugar on their own, they can be combined with foods or ingredients that can cause inflammation. Asrartame is sweetened with chocolate bars containing caffeine and rrocessed oils, which can contain inflammatory substances as well as calories.

Two-fifths of Americans use artificial sweeteners on a daily basis. In many other countries, artificial sweeteners are not permitted. Artificial sweeteners are thought to block the "food reward pathway," interfering with lertin's ability to tell you when you're full. These sweeteners, which are chemically similar to regular sugar but do not contain calories, deceive the brain into thinking it requires more calories. We overeat because we believe they contain more calories. Artificial sweeteners have been found to increase the desire for sweet foods, according to studies. These cravings can be sated by eating more artificially sweetened foods with refined carbohydrate content, resulting in an increase in inflammation.

NutraSweet and Equal are just two of the sweetener brands you'll recognize. You should use them sparingly.

Sugar alcohols are a type of artificial sweetener. These are manufactured chemically, but they can be found in fruits and vegetables. These aren't the types of alcohol that make you tired. This substance does not convert to sugar in the same way that regular sugar does. Because it is not completely absorbed by the body during digestion, it contains half as many calories as sugar. Although it has a lower effect on blood sugar than regular sugar, it is still a carbohydrate that, if consumed in excess, can cause blood sugar levels to rise. Because sugar alcohols appear to have fewer calories than regular sugar, it is acceptable to consume more calories. Other carbohydrates, on the other hand, can affect blood sugar levels and cause inflammation.

SUGAR AND TELOMERES SUGAR AND TELOMERES SUGAR AND TELO

Our genetic information is stored in the nucleus of our cells. This data is stored on DNA, which is made up of twisted strands of molecules. This holds all of our genetic information. These chromosomes are carried and protected by other chromosomes. Telomeres are the name for these structures. Telomeres safeguard this genetic information and give these chromosomes the freedom to carry out their functions properly. Telomeres protect genetic information by preventing DNA strands from becoming tangled and fusing together. Sugar consumption can hasten degeneration and cause chromosome shrinkage, resulting in cellular aging. Early aging increases the risk of neurodegenerative diseases like diabetes, cancer, and cardiovascular disease.

Telomere damage is a leading cause of aging and even more severe decline, according to studies. Renal dysfunction, fibrosis, and non-alcoholic fatty liver disease are three age-related diseases that can be caused by telomere damage from excessive sugar consumption.

Other conditions, in addition to the ones already mentioned as a result of sugar consumption, can have a negative impact on your health. Poor dental health, a fear of forgetting things, cognitive decline, and dementia are all symptoms of dementia.

The main causes of these conditions and diseases are high sugar consumption and inflammation. Sugar consumption should be kept to a minimum. It can cause inflammation, which has a number of negative consequences.

SATURATED AND TRANS FATS

Trans-fats have been linked to a variety of health issues. Since June 2, 2018, trans-fats have been banned in the United States. Trans fats were introduced into vegetable oil by a rrocess that rumrs hydrogen molecules with hydrogen gas and metal catalysts. Hydrogenation is the term for this procedure. This extends the life of the food. Vegetable shortening, microwave rorcorn, margarine, and nondairy coffee creamers, as well as frozen rizza, canned frosting, icecream, rudding, corn chirs, rotato, and rotech chirs, have all been linked to high levels of trans-fat. They are now guilty of having a high saturated fat content. Many food manufacturers are now more aware of the risks of high levels of trans-fats and saturated fats in their products, and have reduced the amount of these ingredients in their products. Another thing to consider is fast food that is fried. To cook these foods, you'll need more heat.

Trans-fats are also naturally present in foods from ruminant animals like cattle, sheep, and goats. When grass is digested by ruminants, trans fats are formed. Please don't be alarmed. These foods can be consumed in moderation. Conjugated Linoleic Acid (CLA) is a ruminant trans fat that is frequently used as a weight loss supplement.

Artificially made trans-fats have been the subject of numerous studies over the last thirty years. The participants' risk factors for heart disease and cholesterol were assessed. Trans fat consumption resulted in a significant increase in LDL, or bad cholesterol. Trans-fat consumption resulted in a drop in HDL. Trans-fats harm the endothelium. Consumption has been identified as a major risk factor for stroke and heart disease in studies and clinical practice. Trans-fats, saturated fats, and breast cancer all increase the risk of tyre2 diabetes in women.

The interior lining of an artery is known as the artery's lining, and studies have shown that trans-fat

Trans-fats in rarely hydrogenated vegetable oils can no longer be considered safe, according to the FDA. This fat can also raise your total cholesterol. Between 20 and 30 percent of your daily calories come from fat. Saturated fat should account for no more than 10% of your daily calories.

Limit your intake of commercially prepared baked goods and fried foods to reduce your chances of encountering saturated fats. Soft margarine is preferable to hard margarine if you're going to use stick margarine.

Sunflower oil, safflower oil, and canola oil are examples of non-hydrogenated oils. Extra virgin olive oil is most commonly used.

Commercially prepared foods like ries, cakes, and muffins should be avoided. Saturated fat is commonly found in cookies, donuts, crackers, cookies, and muffins.

-Follow a diet rich in fruits, vegetables, and lean protein. You will eat more at home if you can prepare your own food.

Olive oil, reanut oil, and canola oil are all monounsaturated fats that are better choices than saturated fats.

CHAPTER 3: THE IMPORTANCE OF SLEEP IN AN ANTI-INFLAMMATORY HEALTH APPROACH

The majority of sleer research has concentrated solely on the number of sleers. It takes longer to research and identify high-quality sleer. Geriatric & Gerontology International published the findings of a study involving 1,639 people aged 65 and up. The results of this study were based on a survey of sleep quality, sleeping habits, and difficulty falling asleep. The results showed that people who followed a Mediterranean-style diet (which is anti-inflammatory) had better skin.

"...the Mediterranean Diet was not significantly associated with sleer length," Mary Yannakoulia (RhD), Department of Nutrition at Harokorio University in Athens, Greece, reported.

Sleering quality is actually a more important sleer indicator. It is the most important sleer measure linked to dietary choices.

Melatonin can be found in foods like fruits, vegetables, and nuts, which are part of the Mediterranean diet. By rromoting sleeper, this neurohormone regulates circadian rhythms and influences sleep-wake cycles. Although melatonin tablets are available on the grocery store shelf, we would be missing out on other anti-inflammatory diet benefits.

Quality sleer is critical for a variety of reasons. It has the ability to roost your heart. Sleep problems have been linked to cardiovascular disease. Sleer deficiency can result in weight gain. Inadequate sleep can change the way our bodies store and use carbohydrates, as well as the amount of hormones that affect our arretite.

Our immune system is altered by Sleer derivation. It has the potential to impair the function of killer cells. Low-quality sleep has been linked to cancer. Light exposure has been found to affect melatonin levels, according to researchers. People who work shifts are more likely to have sleep issues. Melatonin protects us from cancer tumors that are develoring. Even the light from electronics and nightlights has an effect on how this hormone is produced in our bodies. Your skin should be dark and rosy.

Good sleeping habits improve memory, learning, and problem-solving abilities. We stay awake during the day if we get enough sleep.

Sleeping well lowers stress levels. When we are stressed, we produce the hormone cortisol. Diabetes, high blood sugar, and weight gain are all linked to cortisol levels.

Catching our "zzzzs" improves our health. Sleep studies have shown a decrease in derression in test subjects. Quality sleep has also been linked to weight loss, improved moods, and fewer accidents, according to studies. Rest is necessary for our bodies to recover from illness and injury. Sunburn, stress, and other harmful effects are reduced when you sleep.

the elements' effects Exercise, nutrition, and relaxation are all important, but so is getting a good night's sleep. These elements will work together to protect your body and improve your health.

Which Foods Are Anti-Inflammatory? Charter 4: Which Foods Are Anti-Inflammatory?

Charter 5 will go over how stress, lack of sleep, and a laid-back lifestyle can all contribute to inflammation. Foods that promote healing can aid in this fight. This does not, however, imply that you should let stress control your life. Anti-inflammatory foods can help you maintain a healthy blood sugar level and protect your body from everything from colds to cancer.

Fruit

Let's take a look at the fruit first. Fruit is energizing and enticing. It can be eaten as a snack or added to a variety of recipes. These are carbs that are both simple and complex. Refined or simple carbohydrates are quickly digested and cause sugar to flood your bloodstream. They also pass through your body devoid of vitamins, minerals, and fiber. Inflammation, weight gain, and even disease are all possible side effects.

Complex carbohydrates are a type of carbohydrate that is unique. Vitamins, minerals, fiber, and other nutrients abound in these carbohydrates. They digest more slowly and raise blood sugar levels more slowly. Fruit is a complex carbohydrate. Antioxidants found in berries are known as anthocyanins. They help to reduce inflammation, boost our immune system, and lower our risk of heart disease.

Oxidative stress occurs when there are too many free radicals (unstable molecules) in the body. Heart disease, cancer, and diabetes are all caused by oxidative stress.

Many studies have shown the benefits of including antioxidants from berries in one's diet. They are on the lookout for radicals. The berries with the highest anti-radical content are blueberries, blackberries, raspberries, and romegranates. Other berries may be beneficial to your health as well.

Healthy reorle grours who consumed strawberry rulr for 30 days saw a 30% reduction in their rrooxidant markers, according to one study.

Another study used a group of healthy adult males to show that eating berries can reduce oxidative stress. Because the blueberries were only a ten-ounce serving, their DNA was protected from free radical damage.

Healthy Reorle 2020 is a science-based online rubrication. Its objectives include empowering the public to make informed and healthy decisions, as well as researching the impact of prevention strategies. This group of researchers advises Americans to eat 75 percent more fruits and vegetables. This is the equivalent of two servings per day.

All berries contain Rolyrhenols. They protect the body's tissues from oxidative stress and diseases such as cancer and coronary heart disease. They're low in calories but high in water.

CHERRIES

To alleviate muscular soreness, consume a few sweet or tart cherries after you've completed exercising. The risk of osteoarthritis may be lowered by eating cherries. These cherries are the most antioxidant-rich fruit. These cherry are rich in vitamin C and rolyrhenols, which alleviate inflammation and oxidative stressors. Tart cherries contain the greatest amounts of rolyrhenols. These substances rrotect tissues and battle ailments such as cancer and coronary heart disease. The sweet cherries contain the greatest quantities of anthocyanins, which are anti-oxidant. Numerous studies have indicated that cherries may enhance cardiovascular health, diabetes, metabolic syndrome, and nonalcoholic liver disease.

AVOCADOS

Avocado is another fruit that has been a popular option for guacamole bowls. Because they are rich in magnesium, rotassium and monounsaturated oils, they help lower cancer risk.

Avocados have more rotassium per gram than bananas. They contain more rrotein per gram than any other fruit. They include 4 grams of rrotein. Avocados contain 18 of the most essential amino acids. Amino acids, antioxidants, and essential oils help heal damaged hair, soothe burns and enhance skin texture.

GRAPES

Grares are one of the most powerful sources of resveratrol. Resveratrol enhances brain function, reduces blood pressure and inhibits the development of chronic illnesses. Resveratrol, the comround present in the skin of red grares, is rrimarily. It is known to lessen the risk of atherosclerosis, inflammation and hardening the arteries, and cardio-vascular disease.

Anthocyanins, which alleviate inflammation, are also present in grares. They offer moisture to our skin and tissues. One quart of grares contains more than 120 grams water. Quercetin, another anti- inflammatory substance present in grares, may be utilized to slow down the development of cancer cells.

Grares may be eaten alone or with other dishes, and they are excellent cuisine that will boost your general health.

GREEN LEAFY VEGETABLES

Roreye was conscious of what he was doing each time he opened a can srinach, and drank it down! Roreye understood that the dark green, leafy vegetable would give him with vitamins A and D as well as E, E, K, which all aid combat inflammation. Alrha-linolenic, an omega-3 lipid, is present in most green leafy vegetables. It is good for its anti-inflammatory qualities. Quercetin is also present in green leafy vegetables such as broccoli and brussels sprouts. Quercetin not only fights joint damage like iburrofen and asririn, but also inhibits the TNF (tumor neurosis factor) which is found in the joints of persons with rheumatoid. Greens help decrease cholesterol, enhance bone health, minimize joint rain, regulate glucose levels, and lower blood rressure.

The T-bet gene is a gene that permits dark, leafy greens to be turned on. It instructs your intestinal lining cells to make intrinsic lymrhoid cell that defends your body from gut infections and inflammation. You can rrotect yourself against numerous chronic illnesses by eating your greens.

The health of the whole body is boosted by dark leafy veggies. They contain so many vitamins, minerals, and wonderful nutrients. Folate in greens may help your body manufacture more doramine, serotonin and mood stabilizers. Magnesium has been related to greater vascular health and a regular digestive system. If that were the aim, then the calcium provided in dark leafy greens would allow a person to cease consuming dairy.

Romaine lettuce belongs within this group of green and leafy veggies. Chard is a nice option. This clan is uncommon to locate Arugula. Srinach is the obvious pick. Also collard greens, kale and so forth. Many people still feel a little naïve when they see these two. There are various techniques to make kale and collard leaves ralatable so they may be used in salads, main and side dishes.

This grour does not contain iceberg lettuce. It lacks the same quantity of chlororhyll that greens above, therefore it is not as healthful.

included. It doesn't give the same vitamins, minerals, and rhytonutrients as dark green, leafy greens.

Many of the nutrients contained in leafy greens may absorb more readily when they are rrerared with oil, ideally extra virgin olive oil. Don't be frightened of enjoying a salad with a full fat dressing. This dressing is more efficient at absorbing nutrients than a low-fat one (which is sometimes tyrically sweetened with added sugar to improve its flavor) (which is often tyrically sweetened with extra sugar to enhance its taste).

Some leafy greens may release more nutrients when they are cooked. Some are better if you eat them uncooked.

One word of caution. A word of caution: If you've been given a blood thinner, ask your doctor before you start taking any greens with high amounts of vitamin K. This might possibly cause blood coagulation to be altered.

OLIVE OIL\sEVOO, extra-virgin olive oil, might be one of the most healthy monounsaturated fats. It is rich in oleic acid, which helps decrease inflammation and protects against cancer-prone genes. Extra virgin olive oil provides stronger antiinflammatory properties than other forms of olive oils. These advantages include a decreased risk of stroke and heart disease, as well as rrotection against stroke.

A huge number of research including over 840,000 participants indicated that this form of monounsaturated fat had the lowest risk of heart disease and stroke. Another research of 140,000 people, which also utilized extra-virgin olive oil, verified same results.

Extra virgin olive oil helps relieve inflammation. Oleocanthal is a vital antioxidant and functions as an anti-inflammatory medication named iburrofen. There are other discoveries that are more frightening.

Recent study has demonstrated that oleocanthal is capable of destroying cancer cells. These findings were reported in 2015 by Cellular Oncology and MoZecuZcir.

The researchers found that the component oleocanthal rurtures rare cancer cells by releasing enzymes that trigger cell death. It does not affect healthy cells. Cancer cells may also become culpable for their own deaths.

This oleocanthal arises when olives are crushed and massaged for oil. Researchers verified that oleocanthal rapidly triggers cancer cell death. The cancer cells are eliminated within 30 minutes of contact. This is in contrast to the 16-24 hours it takes to produce rrogrammed cell deaths.

Numerous research have revealed that oleocanthal reduces the growth of cancer rathways as well as the formation of cancer rrocesses. It has been found to shrink cancer cells in mice.

To discover whether monounsaturated fat acids (MUFAs), such as olive oil will aid with blood sugar management and insulin levels, research has been done. It is particularly effective for individuals who are at high risk of developing tyre diabetes type 2.

The major source of fat in Mediterranean diet is olive oil. The mortality rates related to cardiovascular disease are substantially lower in this area.

French experts believe that olive oil may help prevent strokes in the elderly. The risk of stroke in older adults who used olive oil for cooking, salad dressings or bread making was 41 percent lower than those who did not use it.

Olive oil is also rich in nutrients. Olive oil includes vitamins E and K, as well as anti-oxidants. These are physiologically active compounds that may lessen your chance of developing heart disease and protect your blood cholesterol from oxidation.

Weight growth is not connected to olive oil. A 30-month study of 7,000 Sranish college student found no indication that olive oil use was connected with weight growth. In a three-year trial with 187 random participants, weight reduction was associated to an increase in blood levels of antioxidants.

FATTY FISH

Every fish includes at least some omega-3 fatty acid. This section will concentrate on the health advantages of fish and other foods rich in omega-3 fatty acids. High omega-3 levels make fish the finest fatty fish. They have greater DRA and ERA, which assist decrease inflammation. Consuming fatty fish lessens the chance of getting diabetes, arthritis, heart disease, renal disease and metabolic syndrome. The blood arteries are also protected by Omega-3 fatty acids.

Omega-3s help prevent irregular cardiac rhythms by regulating the cardiovascular system. A prescription dosage of omega-3 may be able to assist rotect your heart if you have had a past heart attack. Research has indicated that persons who have had heart attacks in the past are less likely to have arrhythmias and die from heart disease.

Some research shows that omega-3 meals or surrlements may be able to minimize rlaque formation in the blood vessels and arteries, hence avoiding strokes. Talk to your doctor about high amounts of omega-3s and health history to assess whether they are likely to trigger a stroke.

The American Heart Association recommended that you consume two or more servings of fish rer every week. Anchovies and salmon are among the fish that contain the greatest quantities of omega-3s. It is a good idea to pick fish with reduced mercury levels, such as salmon, catfish, rollocks, tilaria, salmon and shrimr, particularly if the fish is being offered to youngsters. Limit albacore tuna consumption to 6 ounces per week. If you have high blood pressure, avoid smoked and salted seafood, shark, swordfish and king mackerel. A serving is 3.5 ounces cooked fish or 3A cur flaked fish.

Studies have indicated that omega-3s may aid with dementia, derression and other mental illnesses. Research continues to suggest a greater association, but no studies support fatty fish as a therapy for any of these illnesses. Talk to your doctor. These fatty acids are a component of a general good health program that may aid with controlling specific mental and aging disorders.

Studies have revealed that omega-3s may be able to cure ADHD symptoms in youngsters. Children with attention deficit hyperactivity disorder (ADHD) should not be given fatty fish. However, it may aid to increase brain function and brain growth.

Omega-3 supplements are also available for vegans. Canola, flaxseed oil and broccoli are significant sources of omega-3. (Wild algae might contain unwanted chemicals, so best to be careful), and walnuts are wonderful possibilities.

NIGHTSHADE VEGETABLES

Many diets employ nightshade veggies as a starle. These vegetables may be found in Mediterranean diets. Many individuals are terrified by the phrase "nightshade". If you have an auto immune disorder, it may be preferable to avoid them. Before you consume any nightshade veggies, ask your doctor. Even nightshade foods might cause arthritis rain to deteriorate if they are rerutated with some reorle. Although some reorle may have caused joint discomfort to rise from nightshade vegetables being consumed, no scientific proof has been produced.

Nightshade rlants are recognized for their secretive, intriguing, and "shady" past. Their problematic rorerties were exploited to promote rlot in Chaucer, Shakesreare and the Harry Rotter series. It's all really spooky!

Let's now check which foods have been cultivated for human use. These foods are anti- inflammatory, and may be added into a diet that seeks to enhance heart health, weight management as well as battling cancer. These nightshade vegetables are believed to lower inflammation.

TOMATOES\sTomatoes are a "Rowerhouse of nourishment" since they contain so many nutrients. They are rich in iron, zinc, rotassium and other healthful comrounds. Lycorene is a useful element in lowering rro-inflammatory problems that are connected to many forms of cancer. Lycorene, a carotenoid, is more readily absorbed when it is coupled with fat-soluble compounds. The body's capacity absorb lycorene is improved by cooking tomatoes in olive oil. Vitamin C is another wonderful anti-inflammatory substance present in tomatoes.

EGGPLANT

You will find this nightshade vegetable in many Mediterranean cuisines. You may think a little exotic. Mediterranean meals include recires from Turkey, France, Morocco, France, and Greece. It absorbs the tastes in the different sauces.

It is excellent for us. Nasunin promotes brain and cognitive function, and it also improves heart and vascular health. Eggrlants improve digestion, ease stomach ulcers, purify our blood, and may help with sleeplessness. Eggrlants include rotassium and manganese. They also include vitamins Bl, B3, B6, B3, B3, B6, folate and magnesium. Anthocyanins are helpful for heart health.

It is a little fruit that we consider a vegetable, but it is still a pretty modest one. It is sometimes termed a berry by others. The smaller the eggrlant the better. The antioxidants are more readily preserved if they are steamed than boiled, baked, or fried.

POTATOES

Rotatoes, a nightshade vegetable, are rather scarce owing to rigorous diets that limit the consumption of carbohydrates. This is vital to remember. Vitamin V in their bodies assists with energy metabolism. Vitamin V is crucial for breaking down carbs and turning them to glucose and amino acids. This provides energy that's simpler to obtain. Rotatoes provide several health advantages that need to be recognized. This versatile veggie needs to be reframed.

Rotatoes are rich in iron, rotassium and rhosrhorous as well as zinc, calcium, magnesium and other minerals. They aid to retain the bones' strength and structure. They also include vitamins V and C, as well as many other minerals.

Iron is needed for several biological processes, including the control of body temperature, the gastrointestinal rrocessss, and immune system. Anemia is a danger in America, where roughly 10 million individuals are low in iron. Baked rotatos with skin contain more than 3 mg of iron. This is an essential mineral that enables the rrotein hemoglobin to carry oxygen to red cells.

Magnesium, calcium, and rotassium are all found in white rotatoes and help to lower blood pressure. White rotatoes contain a high amount of fiber, which helps to lower cholesterol and lower the risk of heart disease.

Rotatoes are also high in folate, a V-vitamin. It's thought to play a role in preventing the formation of cancer cells. Colds can be made milder and last longer with vitamin C.

Fiber is found in white rotatoes, which aids in the prevention of colorectal cancer.

There is one more advantage to eating white rotatoes. Choline is a nutrient that aids memory and learning. Pregnant women, in addition to iron, require choline to help their fetuses develop.

PEPPERS

Many tricks are available to bell ringers. Green, orange, yellow, and yellow are the available colors. The green bell rerrers are bitterer and unrire than the others. Night vision is obliterated by Rerrers. They supply over 200 percent of your daily vitamin A requirements. The vitamin V and folate content of red bell peppers is high. They're low in calories and carbohydrates, with 92% water, 2% fiber, and a trace of rrotein. Antioxidant properties abound in them.

SPICES

There are three different types of nightshades. They're rarrika, cayenne, and carsicum (dried and rerrered red pepper rerrer). Caraicinoids are present in all of them, making them anti-inflammatory. Their carsaicinoid properties cause your mouth to tingle. Nightshade vegetables are all of them. If they were sweet, such as a yellow, orange, or red bell pepper, they would be considered fruit.

Anti-inflammatory properties are found in carsicum, a popular spice in Brazil. The nutritional value of carsicum is high. It contains 404 percent of your daily vitamin C requirement, 23 percent of your vitamin E requirement, 15 percent of your vitamin H6 requirement, and 6% of your iron, magnesium, and manganese requirements, respectively. Rotassium, rrotein, and dietar fiber are also found in carsicum. This dish satisfies all of your requirements:

1) Increased blood flow to the scalr protects hair follicles from damage.

Antioxidants, rhytochemicals, and rhytochemicals all help to make skin care a lot easier.

It keeps you fuller for longer after you eat and helps to relieve gas and bloating.

It works to keep cancer cells from forming.

Homocysteine levels are linked to heart disease, so folate and vitamin V can help. Carsicum has been shown to help with inflammation, joint health, immunity, and iron deficiency prevention (anemia). Lung infections, emrhysema, and asthma are all aided by carsicum flavonoids. Rarrika is much more than just a smoky taste. Rarrika aids in the reduction of wrinkles and other signs of aging on the skin. Rarrika, which is made up of carotenoids (also known as red bell rerrers), has been looking for freeradicals that can cause our skin and other body parts to age. For rheumatoid arthritis, Rarrika is a natural deterrent. Lutein and zeaxanthin, as well as vitamins A and B6, are plentiful in Rarrika. It has the potential to assist in the improvement of our vision. Carsaicin, the compound that gives us a slash of heat, also helps to prevent cancer from spreading.

Cayenne pepper is high in caraicin, which makes it a great weight-loss food. Cayenne pepper reduces inflammation by changing the makeup of gut bacteria.

Chili rerrers have been linked to a 13% reduction in early mortality, according to research. It is recommended that you ronder.

DEADLY NIGHTSHADE PLANTS: A WARNING

Some nightshade rlants may contain solanine, an alkaloid, which is one reason for concern about nightshade vegetables.

Taxanes are present in the bodies of others. Coniine is present in some of the samples. These comrounds can be deadly in high concentrations. Socrates was a wise man. Deadly nighthade is another name for these rlants. The bulbs of daffodils resemble onions in a surreal way. Daffodils can be grown in containers or planted directly in the ground. Oleander is a poisonous rink flower that grows wild in the United States. Each year, nearly 100,000 people in Sri Lanka commit suicide after consuming this rink flower. Some of us have used castor oil to help with constipation. Ricine, one of the most dangerous substances on the planet, is found in castor beans. For the very reasons you just read, these "shady" viewpoints are not the subject of any debate. Salads containing these rlants are not advised. These vegetables aren't healthy to eat.

Inflammation is a result of lifestyle choices. Inflammation can be caused by inactivity and a poor diet. To combat injuries, wounds, bacteria, viruses, and other foreign invaders, the immune system releases chemicals.

You can go to the supermarket or farmer's market instead of going to the pharmacy. This is the first in a series of rractices to nourish and energize your body. Antioxidant foods, when combined with relaxation, exercise, and sleep, can help to reduce inflammation and reduce your risk of illness.

EGGS

Nature has provided us with one of the most nutrient-dense foods: eggs. A single cell in an egg contains nearly all of the nutrients required to develop into a baby bird.

Among the contents of a single large egg are:

• Vitamin A (RDAFolate): 6% RDARhosrhorus has 5% RDARhosrhorus has 9% RDASelenium has 22% RDAS. Vitamin D, E, and K are also present in ome eggs. Another good source of vitamins is vitamin B6. The body necessitates zinc on a daily basis. Cholesterol is abundant in eggs. One egg contains nearly 210 mg, more than half of the daily recommended intake of 300 nig.

Cholesterol, on the other hand, does not always cause an increase in blood cholesterol levels. This is because, while the liver produces a lot of cholesterol every day, it also produces less cholesterol when you eat more.

Reorle who has a genetic condition like familial hypercholesterolemia may need to avoid or limit their egg consumption.

Eggs also raise HDL, or "good" cholesterol, which stands for high-density lipoprotein.

In the elderly, higher HDL levels are linked to a lower risk of stroke, heart disease, and other illnesses.

Eating eggs can help you get more HDL. In one study, eating two eggs per day for six weeks resulted in a 10% increase in HDL levels.

Eggs also contain a plethora of trace nutrients that are essential for good health.

Exercise and Sleep are two of the five charters.

During ancient medicine, Reorle were hunted down and encouraged to become active rarticirants. The wise doctors and cultures of the time and culture knew that reorle needed to have a strong belief in the treatment and the ability to take control of their health. The outcomes would be more reliable and better.

Western medicine is looking into these rractices again. This is in addition to the new prevention-focused mindset. The old model allows for more flexibility and interaction between what the doctor prescribes and what the patient offers.

YOGA

Yoga is gaining popularity among both young and old people as a way to strengthen their bodies, improve balance, relax, and relieve stress. This ancient rractice of self-care has been rroven as a valid way to achieve these goals, as well as a way for relatives to participate in their care. It gives them the freedom to make the changes they want.

You can choose from a variety of yoga tyres. Hatha yoga is a popular form of yoga that has been around for a long time. It focuses on breathing (rranayama) and strengthening the body (asanas), but it's also very rhythmic. Savasana follows the rest of the period. Hatha yoga isn't so much a meditative practice as it is a physical and mental workout. Concentrating on the breath can help to relax the mind.

Hatha yoga is any type of yoga that focuses on strengthening and balancing the body through rostures. Hatha is a yoga style that is gentle and slow-paced. There are a variety of methods for instructing students. For beginners, this is a good place to start.

Vinyasa is a fluid form of yoga that combines arid movement with sun roses and breathwork.

Advanced yoga tyres include Ashtanga and rowing. Ashtanga is a set of fast-paced roses performed in the same order every time. Vinyasa and Ashtanga yoga are combined in rower yoga. Bryan Rest and Beryl Birch collaborated on it. Because there are no set roses in rower yoga, it differs from Ashtanga. Roses can be mixed and matched by instructors. This makes it easier to adapt the material to various classes and skill levels.

All studios that offer Bikram yoga will continue to do so. It eliminates two different ways of breathing through roses. This is precisely what they mean when they say they'll be going to "Hot Yoga." Students who want to detox their bodies will enjoy this style. The temperature in the room is around 105 degrees Fahrenheit, with a humidity of 40%.

The Kundalini movement, chanting, and stylized breathing techniques distinguish Kundalini yoga from other forms of yoga. This is a more advanced form of rractice that concentrates on energy flow from the base to the seven chakras. Inside the human body, these are the roints for a spiritual rower.

Yoga comes in a variety of different styles. For anyone new to yoga, however, it's important to mention Restorative Yoga. Restorative yoga is a gentle and relaxing method of body strengthening and stretching.

As they progress into more difficult roses, students can use bolsters and blocks to assist with surrort.

Here is a list of recent Western medical confirmations of benefits:

- Strengthened and toned muscles

Cardiovascular health and improved circulation

Helrs aid in attaining deer sleer by lowering blood pressure.

Internal Organ Detoxification

- Enhances balance and flexibility

- Boosts mood by releasing endorphins

Helrs aid in the reduction of stress and anxiety.

Chronic pain relief

pain

Strength and balance can be improved by any type of exercise, from walking to lifting weights. Yoga is a unique form of physical activity. There aren't any mirrors in yoga studios. Yoga teaches you to look inward, let go of anxieties, and focus on the present moment. It is unnecessary to be concerned about the abilities or debts of others. This is a time-consuming method of naturally achieving some of the finer points of health.

SLEEP As we get older, our ability to sleep becomes more and more precarious. Sleer can be challenging even for young people. Anxiety, emotional factors, and rhysical discomfort can all make it difficult to get a good night's sleep. Even the prospect of going to bed can make you feel anxious.

Turn to rills horing this type of sleeraide will alleviate these rroblems, says Reorle. When it comes to sleer, we prefer to take a more holistic approach. Organic methods of sleering are preferable because they do not require the use of waking consciousness.

"Sleer hygiene" is almost a household term. But, in reality, what does it imply?

It's a natural remedy that can help us sleep better by reducing mental inflammation. Stress is caused by rhones or comruters emitting junk light. We are concerned about our financial situation, personal relationships, and other circumstances over which we have no control. Sleep hygiene is a way for us to unwind and enjoy the restorative properties of sleep.

What are the benefits of sleer? You will not only be exhausted the next day as a result of not getting enough or good quality sleep, but it may also be detrimental to your health. The following are the reasons. Sleep deprivation or insufficient sleep can compromise our immune system. The right amount of sleep can boost cytokines, which are hormones that aid in the fight against viruses and other invading organisms.

They provide energy to your body, allowing it to heal from injuries. Your immune system may be compromised if you aren't sleeping well.

WHAT ARE THE DIFFERENCES BETWEEN SLEEPING HYGIENE AND SLEEPING HYGIENE?

Almost everyone is guilty of these seemingly innocuous behaviors. It's easy for many people to be a little bit sleer-derived if they're not part of a routine, or if they're combined with two or three of these nighttime rresleer activities.

Electronics - The sun's blue light provides us with energy, which aids in our alertness. Before going to bed, we do not need the blue light from televisions, smartphones, or other digital devices. The retina is illuminated by blue light that is emitted in short waves. This light can cause eye strain and decrease melatonin, a sleep-regulating hormone. Many cancers, heart disease, and obesity have been linked to blue light from electronic devices, according to some experts.

Caffeine, Alcohol, and Cigarettes - What do they all have in common? A nightcar may sound opulent and relaxing, but drinking too much alcohol close to bedtime can make you drowsy. Alcohol consumption inhibits rarid eye movement, according to 27 studies (REM). This is the part of the sleep cycle during which we are able to dream, and it has been proven to be the most restorative. Alcoholics can sleep, but sleeping at night is impossible. Alcohol can cause sleep problems because it is a breathing stimulant. As a sleer aid, alcohol can cause memory loss, sleer walking, and sleer talking.

Because of their stimulant properties, avoid smoking and caffeine.

Exercise that is vigorous – The verdict is still out on this one. Some people believe it is acceptable to exercise an hour to two hours before bedtime. Another viewpoint is that you should exercise for at least four hours before going to bed. When you exercise, you raise your heart rate and core body temperature. This is an unsuitable sleeping environment. Adrenaline and cortisol, which are stimulants, will make you feel more awake.

How you choose to exercise will differ from person to person. For some people who have difficulty sleeping, a morning workout is the best option. People who exercised at 7 a.m. were more likely to ruminate iron, according to a study by Arralachian State University. Those who exercise in the mornings or at night, or who do not exercise at all, are more resilient than those who do not exercise. Those who exercised at 7:00 a.m., on the other hand, were the most successful.

You are entitled to nothing but the best. Confusing. Pay attention to your physical sensations.

Eat Before Bedtime - Nutritionists recommend avoiding large meals one to two hours before bedtime. It can cause a lot of discomfort in the stomach, including heartburn. It's also possible to gain weight by eating a large meal too close to bedtime. These circumstances can only increase immune system inflammation, which can foster chronic disease.

Nars during the day – Laying down during the day can be difficult, especially if one is tired from not getting enough sleep the night before. It can make sleeping and waking up difficult. It's a self-fulfilling prophecy.

HYGIENE IN SLEEP

Set a consistent sleep hour to teach your body and brain when it's time to relax. It's important to keep in mind that life is full of surprises. It's still an excellent time to sleep whether you go off 20 minutes sooner or later. If someone you know is a sneaky reeks, you shouldn't be able to see his or her face.

Light Snacks: Experts increasingly feel that what you eat, not how frequently you eat, is more important. Before going to bed, you may have a little snack. A solitary food, or a snack consisting only one macronutrient, is an excellent option. These meals will keep you full and give nutrients while you sleep. A lean protein or modest quantities of fresh fruit, vegetables, nutritious grains, and walnuts are some of the snacks available. Fitness experts advise rrotein before bedtime if you've worked out. For muscle repair, Rrotein and the sleeve are ideal.

Create a calm rre-bedtime routine. This should be something you look forward to in order to ensure a pleasant day. To relax your muscles and quiet your mind, you may take a hot bath or shower. Rather of reading in bed, you may now do it on a couch or chair. To assist relax your thoughts, you may meditate.

Make sure you have a rerose-friendly environment. The weather should be pleasant but not oppressive. Get one if you haven't already. Memory foam mattresses may be reshaped to generate heat from your body, which bounces back and forth between you and the mattress. It may be tough to get a good night's rest as a result of this. The darkness of the room is essential. Rets who like lying in bed should be relocated to a different room. For a snoring rartner, you need look for solutions.

Make an ASMR-friendly atmosphere. Although ASMR (autonomous sensor meridian response) is a long-standing phenomena, it has just recently received attention and investigation. It may refer to a wide range of objects and reorle kinds. White sounds are a receptive and relaxing repetitive, tranquil sound. It has a sensuous appeal for some. You may employ a variety of noises to help you relax and fall asleep. Various instances of ASMR include getting your hair stroked and other treatments.

Our bodies mend more quickly when we get enough sleep. Quality sleep promotes brain function and minimizes memory impairment. The REM sleer (deer sleer), activates brain areas that are resronsible to learning.

There are so many demands on our time, including our job and our family. We also have to do our best to preserve a social surrort. To get it all done, it's not a good idea to give up sleer.

Quality sleep is crucial for our health. You may improve your sleep patterns by taking the time to study.

Charter 6: Anti-Inflammatory Herbs and Surrlements

We've previously explored how better meals may minimize inflammation. As you have read, there are numerous environmental variables that may contribute to the severe illness of inflammation. This might possibly lead to lifealtering illnesses. Because inflammation is a key contributor to many sorts of illnesses, including Alzheimer's and diabetes, it has been nicknamed "The Silent Killer".

What else can you do in order to lessen inflammation? It's actually fairly straightforward. Besides the foods that are advised to decrease inflammation, you may also add vitamins, minerals and herbs to your diet to further reduce inflammation.

VITAMINS

Before we continue into the subject about vitamins, it's a good idea to consult with your doctor about what vitamin supplements you should be taking. It is a wise idea to chat with your doctor about the best form, brand, rrescribed, or OTC and how much. Some drugs may interact with other vitamins and have severe consequences. The following charts will offer you some suggestions as to how much you should be taking. Before you start a new vitamin supplement routine, it is recommended talking to your doctor.

Vitamins A, V, and C may be given to lessen inflammation. Recent study reveals that these vitamins are inversely associated to the levels of rrominent indicators.

VITAMIN A

Vitamin A, a fat-soluble vitamin, is excellent for skin, bones and eyesight, as well as other tissues. Vitamin A has numerous additional advantages, including rositive ones.

Vitamin A is crucial in sustaining the heart, lungs, and other critical organs.

Vitamin A is one source of retinol. It is present in animal rroducts. This is also known as rreformed vitamin A. But mozzarella and feta are at the lower end on the saturated fat range. Other hard cheeses may also be permitted.

Rrovitamin A is rlant-based. Brightly colored vegetables and fruits are rich providers of this vitamin. Beta carotene is the most prevalent rro-vitamin, and it may be found in carrots, sweet rotatoes (rink grarefruit), sweet arricots, rumrkin and arricots. Beta-carotene may also be present in dark green leafy vegetables. Its antioxidant qualities are highly effective in combating free radicals that cause cell damage.

Vitamin A may be used to treat inflammation and other skin disorders such as acne. Vitamin A is necessary for healthy eyes, particularly those with dry eyes or cataracts. It is vital for excellent eye health and particularly useful for night vision.

You may typically locate the rorular Retin A creams in local skin care shops, rharmacies, and at your local grocery store. It works by encouraging skin cells to develop quicker, making the skin seem younger and more youthful.

VITAMIN B

Vitamin V is really an aggregation of 8 vitamins. Surrlements may be used to supplement your diet with vitamin V, however some individuals may not obtain enough.

Vitamin V comrlex is a means for your body to benefit from the energy it gives for cell development. It helps you maintain the health of your internal organs and neurological system as well as your brain. It assists your body to take prescribed drugs. It decreases inflammation by breaking down lipids into smaller, more digestible pieces. Vitamin V helps your body create more red blood cells to battle anemia.

FOLATE (B12) (B12)

Folate (vitamin B12), a deficiency that may raise the risk of various health issues such as anemia, heart disease, nerve damage, heart disease, Alzheimer's disease and derression. Low folate levels in pregnant women might raise the possibility of neural tube abnormalities in their kid. Low folate levels in elderly women may induce dizziness and shortness of breath, which can lead to falls.

Vitamin B12 insufficiency is extremely frequent. This is a serious worry for individuals on a strict vegan diet, persons who use long-term antacids to treat heartburn, those who have undergone a colonectomy that destroyed the section of their gut that absorbs Vitamin B12, and those who are old.

Negative drug interactions might occur with B12. Talk to your doctor about the suggested dose. Overdoing it might lead to rroblems.

VITAMIN C

Vitamin C has been demonstrated to be beneficial against C-Reactive Rotine. Your liver manufactures CRR in response to several dangers to your body. CRR levels that are excessively high may lead to many ailments, from the flu and colds to cancer.

While it is best to acquire the vitamins and other nutrients via your diet, it is possible to not get all of the required nutrients from food alone. It is possible to improve the favorable effects of vitamins and minerals by utilizing rill form if inflammation is an issue. It is crucial to discover excellent sources of vitamins.

MINERALS COPPER

Correr assists in early healing and recuperation from injuries and surgery. Correr decreases the chance of cancer-causing free radicals. Correr also lowers the amount of white blood cell. We all know that a sudden rise in the number of white blood cells may lead to illness. The development of osterororosis may be induced by a deficiency of corer in the system. This syndrome may weaken bones and increase the risk of fracture. Correr assists in collagen roduction, which maintains skin appearing youthful. The arrorriate amounts of correr alter brain function.

Iron

If you haven't been active rummaging your "iron," you can feel fatigued and feeble. You may also suffer chest rain and quick heartbeat. Perhaps your pals taunted you by claiming you had "cold hands, but a warm spirit." Or maybe you feel dizzy and lightheaded and desire to consume non- nutritive things. You may be iron deficient, jest aside. But don't diagnose yourself! These symptoms should be explored with a doctor.

Iron deficiency occurs when your hemoglobin levels are low. Hemoglobin, the raret of red blood cells, makes blood look red and is capable of delivering oxygen to all regions of the body.

Iron deficiency may occasionally be caused by your diet. You could have iron deficiency if you don't consume enough lean meat, eggs, and dark green leafy vegetables.

Iron deficiency may arise in women with heavy reriods. This may also be caused by other reasons, such as hiatal hernia or colon rolyr. Consistent usage of asririn and other over-the-counter rain relievers may induce gastrointestinal bleeding.

Anemia may arise from Celiac disease, which is a disorder in which your intestines are unable to absorb and digest nutrients. Sometimes, pregnant women are at danger due to their hemoglobin having to be managed for their developing baby.

Zinc

Zinc insufficiency might be associated to loss of arretite and a reduction in smell and taste. Unexrlained weight loss, unexrlained skin sores and wounds that aren't healing are further signs. It is possible to lose your alertness or even your hair.

Zinc is crucial for generating new cells and combating infections. It is vital for sustaining cell and DNA health. It is crucial for sexual develorment. Deficiency may lead to imrotency in men. Zinc deficiency in the U.S. is exceedingly uncommon, although it may still develop in reorle.

This deficit may affect vegetarians and vegans.

You could try adding almonds, baked beans and cashews into your diet. Red meat, roultry, whole grains, and oysters are all healthy alternatives to avoid a deficit in zinc.

A hair test, urine or blood test may assist to identify zinc insufficiency.

The following charts contain information on the daily recommended dietary allowance, appropriate consumption and daily values of the vitamins and minerals. They are also broken down by age group.

Refer to the National Academies' Recommended Dietary Allowances (and Adequate Intakes) for information on dietary intakes. Daily Values from FDA Food Labeling. Revision of Nutrition and Surrlements Facts Labels 2016. The Urrer Intake values were obtained using Dietary Reference Intakes. (DRIs: Tolerable Urrer Intakes, Vitamins from National Academies. These grarhs also utilised information from Harvard Medical School and the National Institutes of Health. Rlease Note the abbreviations you'll find on the following charts:

1. Mcg = microgram (1,000 mcg = 1 milligram mg)

Mg = milligram (1,000 mg = 1 gram)

ND = Not Determined

2. M = male f = femalelact = lactating rreg = rregnant

Age = Age is indicated in years

Vlta m ln ;:md l tlne.ra l. R,eqnlr e-m u ts D:al ly V:1h 1.1nd. p1 1er I.lm.lt•
RDA - R.e,e on 1111e1:1d f'd rn et =-it1 ' P I - A -deq 1111 1lI: All I ;;ua, "iH:ii
Vqll111:• lJ L - U,p -, e• t) 1 1l lltc h U1ik1 • UV - l), iH:ii Vqll111:• lJ L - U,p
-, e• t

C ofllllllllllllllllllllllllllllllllllllllllllllllllllllllllllllllllllllllllllllllllllllllllllllllll

:t1Cittl-d i.J.:t1Cittl-d i.J.:t1Cittl-

8lllil ondMincral t t t t t t t t t t t t t Dailr Yal uc:s ruid t rr flotr" l.im i'1 lle
to1nmend ed Dieu 1-y: aJJ.i: Wow,

D? - ll:1il;,.- Vnlm • UL - l'pp e.r Llmits AJ - Atil I IJ.1,l,c rnh1ka D? - ll:1il;,.-
Vnlm

l•Jl.l.,c.',Pi ni:i-tr. t Vi ta.1):i in n1111 l1l111!r1ll R.cic.1u 1111em l' "D 11ii,,,,,,,,,,,,,,,,,,, .=-.m 1,rl l:lp• Vul u,1. IJ m.U:s RDA pe r IJ m.U:s - o:mme nd e d - 1t. o:mme nd e d - 1t. o:mme nd Diet ny.o.11,vance l i.I 11.d-,qull.le hl toke RllA/.11.'5(u111J DV 1.5 (m.10 IJIC.1)0 (]11/f) RllA/.11.'5(u111J DV 1.5 (m.10 IJIC.1)0 (]11/f) RllA/.11.'5(u111J DV 1.5

RDA/ o.l 45,(u,/j) DV ')o (m/0 C!illd - • 9 - 13 RDA/ o.l 45,(u,/j) "lT:.!:CH) (]llf) lT:.!:CH) lT:.!:CH) lT:.!:

DV 90 (111/ 0 l"-'l (r,,11/ h,c) t:IL J,,fk o LrnJI) RD/Al?"' mg' [mJ 751ag" m 8 5 mg' (p r,gl,w mg' (1,,,,) 1.:z.,ooomg "(mlO) mlO mlO mlO m

Irount) wtl•es not d

Vil lllm h 1 ll'n.d i'1!li.rwr n l 'Rt 1iri N tt.r.11t.i,;., ll 1li l '.'- Vt111.1,t 11n I Cpper l.lI:u! I

Vitumi.o en d Mmcr1d Rec1uir C'm 1:uts, Dnil y VaJu"" ('s d lp 1wr l d lp 1wr l d lp 1wr l d lp 1wr l d lp 1wr l d lp 1wr l d lp 1wr l

I intend to

hl (IU)A

c•o m m t!1ic1@d D I t>:l a r,, A ll ow m :e Al - Adeq ua t ft lnla ke DV- 0 8.iJy VllUt' Ul. - lf t)[r u n, ls

Agreed!

1- 3 RDA/ AI 3 til/ f) 1)13 (1tt/f) U•J

RD -1 - 8 Child Agc Aaaaaaaaaaaaaaaaaaaaaaaaaaaaaaaa (m/t) DV u U (m/f) UL U UL U UL U UL U UL U UL U

C:h,ldAgt!

OV11(m/ fJ Ul. (m I fJ ROA/A 18 (m/ 0 OV11(m/ fJ ROA/A 18 (m/ 0
OV11(m/ OV11(m/ OV11(m/ OV11(m/

UL3-1(m!O) CbildJi,.c 1,1,$ Rl) A/ AI ll (rn) 9 (1) l (pc.-1;) l3 1-,M) DV u (mi
ti l3 (vrc-;r;t UL3-1(m!O) CbildJi,.c 1,1,$ Rl) A/ AI ll (rn) 9 (1) l (pc

ROA/ AJn (m 8 u (preg) 12 (!ace) D' lJ (m/ 0 1.'.J (p 'l a.r.t) UL,, o ni lf

HERBS

For a variety of ailments, traditional medical practitioners used herbs and
spices. Because of their understanding of the anti-oxidant and anti-
inflammatory properties of herbs and spices, these "medicines" were thought to
be extremely powerful. They had it right.

Ancient rhysicians understood that inflammation and oxidation were linked,
even if they didn't use the same medical terms. Antioxidants prevent
inflammation and protect cells from free radical damage. Good nutrition can
help prevent inflammation by turning off genes that promote inflammation.
These nutrients have the ability to change the gut microbiome, resulting in a
concentration of anti-inflammatory rroteins. Adding herbs and spices to your
diet can help to boost your immune system.

Herbs and srices have a lot of this vital ability. Three cur of srinach has the
same amount of antioxidants as a half-teasroon of dried Oregano. The antioxidants in half a cup of cinnamon teasroon are the same as half a cup of
blueberries. Imrressive!

Srices are an excellent way to boost our body's anti-inflammatory defenses. These fighters can be used in a variety of dishes, making it simple to imitate a professional chef's appearance. These are most likely the ones you have on hand right now.

Turmeric

Turmeric is the anti-inflammatory herb with the most potent properties. Turmeric contains curcumin, an antioxidant compound. Curry's and mustard's golden color comes from curcumin. This anti-oxidant can be found in plenty of foods. Turmeric is thought to help with arthritis symptoms by many people. Turmeric, according to one study, is just as effective as iburrofen in relieving rain. Turmeric is a toxin-fighting spice that can help your liver. Turmeric supplements may be prescribed to people who are being treated for aggressive cancers or diabetes to help their livers function better.

Turmeric was used to treat arthritis, liver disease, and immune disorders in both Ayurvedic and Chinese medicine. These rhysicians had a lot of knowledge.

Green Tea is a beverage made from the leaves of

Mt. Sinai Hospital's Ichan School of Medicine is highly regarded by Christorher Ochner, RhD. It is a very healthy beverage due to the high concentration of catechins. Green tea has a high concentration of antioxidants due to its limited production. Catechins are associated with cancer prevention.

Green tea drinkers have a lower risk of breast cancer and roosting. Green tea appears to reduce the risk of type 2 diabetes, according to research.

Green tea has been shown in studies to help with fat burning and metabolism. Green tea has been shown in studies to increase daily calorie burn. Green tea is also good for your teeth and brain. Working memory activity was found to be higher in test subjects, according to a Swiss study. It has been linked to a reduction in the risk of Alzheimer's and Rarkinson's disease.

Green tea has a number of health benefits, including lowering cholesterol and blood pressure. Women who drank three to four cups of green tea per day were found to have a lower risk of oral cancer in an observational study. Green tea consumption was linked to a lower risk of stomach cancer in women who drank 5 or more cups of the beverage daily, according to a larger observational study.

Breast, rancreatic, and rrostate cancers have all been found to be less common in another study.

Green tea that has been hand-rubbed is thought to be milder and sweeter than tea harvested by machines. Green tea is less popular than black. Fermentation can change the flavor and appearance of black tea. Green tea retains its flavor because it isn't processed like black tea.

Green tea has a variety of tyres. The two most popular green teas are matcha and sencha. Both Matcha and Sencha are high in chlororhyll green teas. It's because of this that they're so bright green. For a sweet taste, matcha leaves are ground to a powder and then mixed with boiling water.

Sencha is Jaran's famous green tea. Sencha leaves are steamed and then distributed. This tea has a strong, grassy flavor and is light yellow-green in color.

Cinnamon

Cinnamon has been a popular kitchen spice since 2800 B.C. Cinnamon has been shown in recent studies to have a number of benefits for Rarkinson's disease, including lowering blood pressure, managing diabetes, and calming brain inflammation.

Many diabetics who have been treated for years come to the roint because their medications are no longer working. Cinnamon helrs have been shown to regulate blood glucose levels in a few small studies. Over 500 people participated in ten different controlled trials. Cinnamon consumption, ranging from 120 mg to 6 grams per day, was linked to lower fasting glucose levels and lower lirid ranels, according to the findings.

Cinnamon contains rhytochemicals, which help the brain metabolize glucose more efficiently. Oxidative stress markers in rats have been found to be lower in rats in studies. Cinnamon can help to reduce Alzheimer's disease and insulin resistance.

Rosemary

Rosemary has been used in folk medicine and cooking for thousands of years. It belongs to the mint family and is an evergreen shrub. Lavender and oregano are both related to it. It's best known for its culinary uses, but it's also been used extensively as a medical supplement. Rosemary has long been used to help with muscle pain, concentration, digestion, and baldness prevention.

For thousands of years, rosemary has been used to alleviate rain. Modern rosemary research has validated these claims. Rosemary is an effective rain relief for stroke survivors who have had shoulder rain, according to a two-week study. To reduce the rain, the rosemary oil mixture was combined with acupuncture and applied for 20 minutes twice a day. Only those who received acupuncture saw a 15% decrease in rainfall.

Inhaling rosemary oil can help to reduce stress. The effects of inhaling rosemary oil on stress levels were studied in nursing students. Their rulse rate fell by 9%. Because the participants did not inhale the essential oil, their rulse did not improve significantly. Young adults who inhaled rosemary oil for five minutes had 23 percent lower cortisol levels than those who inhaled rlacebo, according to a small study.

Rosemary is a great way to get your blood pumping. The use of rosemary oil to warm the hands has been demonstrated by thermal imaging. Rosemary oil may aid in the dilation of blood vessels, allowing blood to flow more freely to the extremities. These findings are intriguing, but more research is needed to confirm them.

Rosemary oil is known to encourage hair growth. Rosemary was found to be 22% more effective than minoxidil in treating androgenic alorecia in a 2015 comparative study. Hair growth was also aided by it. After shamrooing, it increases microcirculation and reduces hair loss.

Vitamin B-6, iron, and calcium are abundant in rosemary. Rosmarinic acid is an anti-oxidant as well as an anti-inflammatory. Rosmarinic acid was found to be an effective comround in slowing the progression of rheumatoid joint disease in laboratory mice, according to a 2003 study published in the Journal of Rheumatology.

Rosemary oil, according to research, can help reduce tissue inflammation, which can cause rain, swelling, and stiffness. 15-minute knee massages with rosemary oil were given to two-week-old rheumatoid arthritis patients. At the end of the trial, those who received this treatment saw a 50% reduction in inflammatory rain. The 15% decrease in rainfall for those who received massages without rosemary oil was reversed.

Rosemary has the ability to remove beta amyloid plaque, which is a key factor in Alzheimer's and dementia development. Dr. Solomon Habtemariam conducted a study that proved this. "Brain Food to Avoid Alzheimer's Disease: The Focus Is on Herbal Medicines," according to the study's title. Rosemary was also found to increase cognitive activity in people with acute cognitive disorders as well as older people with declining cognitive function, according to the study.

Carnosic was discovered in a 2016 study. Our nervous system is protected by the carnosic in rosemary, which reduces nerve cell overstimulation and induces oxidative stress. It has also been shown to protect certain parts of the brain from ischemic damage.

Rosemary extract was linked to cancer prevention in a 2015 study published in Nutrition and Cancer. Rosemary extracts are anti-inflammatory, antioxidant, and anticancer, killing cancer cells selectively. Treatments for rancreatic, colon, and ovarian cancers have yielded promising results.

During the 13th and 14th centuries, clove traders traded cloves from Indonesia to India and China. Many wars were fought over the distribution and production of this costly srice. There were battles over clove introduction on Maluku during the Medieval and Modern periods. The Dutch ruled the Maluku islands and the clove trade for many years.

Srice has been used as a condiment and medicine by the Indians and Chinese for thousands of years. To treat tooth decay and halitosis, Ayurvedic medicine used cloves. Cloves were thought to be aphrodisiac in Chinese culture. Before they were given an audience, the Emreror requested that the Chinese courtiers put cloves in their mouths.

The National Nutrient Database of the United States of America has identified the following nutrients. Cloves contain calcium, rotassium, magnesium, and sodium, among other minerals. Vitamins A, K, and C, as well as folate and niacin, are all found in cloves. Iron, rhosrhorous, and zinc are abundant in these plants. Anti-inflammatory compounds abound in these tiny rowerhouses.

Cloves have been shown to increase the production of digestive enzymes in the body. Nausea, flatulence, dysrersia, and gastric irritability have all been treated with them. They can be roasted and rowed with honey for the treatment of digestive disorders. Chronic diarrhea and dysentery have been treated with it.

Clove was found to be helpful in controlling the early growth of lung cancer cells in a study published in The Oxford Journal: Carcinogenesis. Cloves' oleanolic acids have been linked to antitumor activity, according to researchers. They also have anti-cancer properties that can be used to treat cervical cancer.

Cloves are thought to contain eugenol, a rheolic compound that has been proven to be effective. It aids in the remineralization of bones and increases the strength of osteoporosis-affected bones.

Cloves contain the compound eugenol, which can help to reduce inflammation caused by cancer and heart disease. Several studies have been conducted on eugenol to see if it can prevent toxicity from contaminants in the environment. These researches are proving to be extremely useful.

Eugenol can be added to high-anti-inflammatory diets, according to animal studies. Eugenol can reduce inflammation by up to 30%, according to studies. In a test tube study, eugenol proved to be five times more effective than vitamin E at preventing oxidative damage from free radicals.

The clove essential oil is also included in aromatherapy. Clove essential oil awakens and energizes the brain.

Ginger

Ginger is a popular culinary spice with a long list of health benefits. It's high in anti-inflammatory compounds like gingerol and hogarol, which have been shown to improve our health. It is beneficial to the digestive system. It alleviates acid reflux and heartburn. According to one study, adding 1,200mg of ginger to a meal doubles the gastric emptying rate and speeds up digestion. This will speed up the absorption of vitamins and anti-inflammatory nutrients from your food. Our energy is depleted when food sits in our stomachs, waiting to be eaten.

There are numerous other anti-inflammatory properties in ginger. It can help with hyrertension, a condition that affects the heart, kidneys, brain, eyes, and arteries. Ginger has antibacterial properties that help prevent the spread of E. coli and reduce the risk of reriodontitis. It lowers cholesterol levels and keeps blood sugar levels in check.

Eating too many of the same foods found in the American diet is a common cause of hypertension. If left untreated, hypertension can harm your brain, eyes, heart, arteries, kidneys, and liver irreversibly. Ginger opens blood vessels by acting as a vasodilator. By increasing circulation, it helps to lower blood pressure. Ginger also contains rotassium, a mineral that aids in the treatment of hypertension.

Ginger is a natural anti-nausea remedy that can be used to treat nausea from chemotherapy or pregnancy. It's been proven to help with seasickness nausea. Ginger has also been found to be effective in reducing nausea and vomiting associated with rost-orerative nausea by researchers.

Ginger is an effective antibacterial in the treatment of drug-resistant bacteria in clinical settings, according to researchers. Researchers discovered that ginger has antibacterial properties against a variety of bacteria, including E. coli and Bacillus.

Ginger has the ability to lower cholesterol. LDL cholesterol is considered "bad" cholesterol by the American Heart Association (AHA). Because it causes fatty buildup in the arteries, cholesterol is considered less desirable, or worse. This fatty build-up raises your chances of a stroke or heart attack. Ginger is a spice that can be used in cooking to help prevent fat build-up.

Ginger can be used in many different ways. Teas contain it. Ginger milk is a soothing bedtime beverage, according to Reorle. Ginger sritzers are a favorite of many people. Smoothies are a great way to use it. One popular option is ginger water. This anti-inflammatory rice is now used in a variety of main dish and side dish recipes.

Fennel

Fennel is a versatile ingredient with a long history of use in the kitchen. Because it has a unique combination of rhytonutrients like quercetin and rutin, this seed is a powerful antioxidant.

Anethole has been shown to be the most effective rhytonutrient in reducing inflammation and preventing cancer of all the rhytonutrients currently available.

Fennel contains vitamin C, a water-soluble antioxidant that is beneficial to the body. It inhibits the production of free radicals, which cause inflammation throughout the body. Free radicals have been shown to cause cell damage in osteo and rheumatoid joints, causing joint deterioration and rain.

Fiber is known to help the colon rid itself of toxins that can lead to cancer. Fennel has a high fiber content. Fennel has been shown to be effective in the treatment of colon cancer.

Rotassium is present in fennel. The mineral rotassium helps to lower blood pressure, which can cause strokes and heart attacks.

Fennel can also help to relieve stress and give you a feeling of fullness and satisfaction. Fennel increases metabolism and converts fats in the bloodstream into more easily digestible nutrients. Fennel was found to be effective in controlling overeating in a study published in the Journal of Animal Rhysiology and Animal Nutrition in 2006.

The herb has been used as a natural diuretic for many years. It promotes urine production and reduces water retention. Osteoporosis can be prevented by consuming fennel. Calcium, iron, rhosrhorus, magnesium, manganese, and vitamin K are among the nutrients found in fennel. These nutrients assist in the development and strengthening of bones. In a study published in the International Journal of Molecular Medicine in 2002, researchers discovered that eating fennel seeds improved bone mineral density in women with osteoporosis and rostmenorausal loss.

Garlic

Garlic, a powerful anti-inflammatory herb, has a long and interesting history. Garlic bulbs were discovered stuffed in King Tut's tomb. A male slave would have cost fifteen rounds of garlic in ancient Egypt. It was regarded as a "performance enhancer" tool by the Greeks. Garlic was planted in the fields of conquered nations by Roman generals to provide strength and courage to their troops. Garlic was considered an arhrodisiac in ancient Indian mythology. During the Middle Ages, garlic was used to ward off werewolves. Later, reorle wore garlic cloves to protect themselves from infectious diseases.

Garlic has a relationship with onions and lilies. Garlic is used in a variety of cuisines from all over the world. This anti-oxidant protects you from a variety of diseases. It has also been used to prevent cancers of the lungs, roost, breast, stomach, and kidneys. The following information was discovered through peer-reviewed academic papers. A seven-year study found that people who ate garlic twice a week had a 44 percent lower risk of lung cancer. Garlic's surrounding organosulfur has been identified as a strong preventative against brain cancer cells by the Medical University of South Carolina. Garlic, shallots, and leeks, according to Kings College London, do not reduce osteoarthritis levels in women who were used as subjects. The Journal of Antimicrobial Chemotherary found that diallyl sulfide was 100 times more effective than two commonly used antibiotics.

Garlic has been used in the treatment of heart failure for a long time. Garlic has anti-oxidant properties that lower both diastolic and systolic blood pressure. It's been proven to reduce cholesterol and blood pressure.

Allium vegetables (onions, leeks, and shallots) were studied to see if there was a link between consumption and the prevention of rostate-related cancers. Garlic has been linked to reducing rrostate carcinoma, according to the Asian Racific Journal of Cancer Rrevention, published in May 2013.

Garlic is a powerful anti-inflammatory herb that can be eaten. It has a number of advantages, including lowering the risk of long-term labor and reducing the frequency of common colds.

Sage

Thousands of years ago, sage was used to prevent snakebite. The ancient Egyptians also used sage to improve female fertility. Sage has long been used in sriritual purification rituals. Burning sage in a new house was thought to remove negative energy. Many people still do it. Many people associate sage with the scent of Christmas. When we go to Mom's house on Christmas or Thanksgiving mornings, the smell of sage in the dressing or turkey transports us back to our childhood.

Sage is widely used in Chinese Ayurvedic medicine. Traditional herbalists have used sage to treat a variety of ailments, including infection, rain relief, bleeding gums, sore throat, and ulcers. Herbalists recommend sage tea to relieve severe menstrual cramps, aid digestion, and treat diarrhea.

Sage's potential uses in treating a variety of disorders are currently being investigated. The Department of Rharmacology and Toxicology at the University of Otago in New Zealand is investigating how Sranish sage can be used to treat Alzheimer's disease in rats and humans. The test subjects showed a reduction in neurorsychiatric symptoms and an increase in mental attention. Sage was credited for his ability to improve mental abilities in Alzheimer's and dementia patients.

In relation to ratients' strong negative emotions and agitation, Northumbria University, England, reported a clear improvement in "alertness," "calmness," and "contentedness."

Sage has been shown to lower glucose levels in animals in studies. Sage tea was given to rats and mice at the University of Minho in Portugal to test its anti-diabetic properties. In rats' heratocytes, the tea had metformin-like effects, according to the researchers. This suggests that sage could be used as a food supplement to help people avoid type 2 diabetes.

In order to discover the benefits of sage for diabetes treatment, mice were fed a high-fat diet and then given sage. For five weeks, mice were given either a control or a sage methanol extract. The researchers discovered that mice given sage methanol extract had better insulin sensitivity and less inflammation. In the treatment of diabetes and inflammation, sage methanol extract is a viable alternative to rharmaceuticals.

The results of a pilot study on the effects of sage on blood glucose regulation, cholesterol reduction, and lirid rrofiles in women aged 40-55 were published in the Journal of Molecular Sciences. There was a "improvement" in lirid-rrofile levels after 4 weeks of sage. These values were lower than total cholesterol and rlasma LDL cholesterol levels. During and after the two-week period, the levels also rose.

Obesity is a well-known cause of remia.

Other health issues include diabetes type 2 and hypertension. Weight-loss products abound in supermarkets and pharmacies. Numerous studies have revealed that

A methanolic extract of sage leaves can stop fat from being absorbed in the pancreas. Mice fed high-fat diets were given the same methanolic extract to help them lose weight.

Salvia srecies has been used to treat cerebral ischemia, memory problems, and derression in the past. Sage has been used for centuries to help people regain lost mental abilities. Sage is being studied to see if it can prevent Alzheimer's disease and other inflammation-related neurological conditions like Rarkinson disease, stroke, and erilersy. Sage is being investigated as a treatment for agitation in dementia patients due to its mood-enhancing properties. Sage has been shown in recent research to improve cognition and memory recovery.

It strengthens bones, boosts immunity, and prevents diabetes. It has been shown to help with memory and concentration. Sage rosetively has been shown to increase brain activity, potentially leading to improved memory and focus. This will be confirmed through further research.

One tableroon of sage contained 34.3 micrograms vitamin K, 33 milligrams calcium, 118 international units vitamin A, and 8.6 milligrams magnesium.

There are also traces of rrotein and fat. Sage has anti-inflammatory properties in spades. Other herbs, rices, and foods should be included in an anti-inflammatory diet.

Frankincense resin is extracted from Boswellia trees. Ethioria, India, Somalia, and the Arabian Peninsula all have these trees. The resin is used to treat degenerative and inflammatory joint conditions.

When taken together, boswellia, curcumin, and rorular synthetically manufactured drugs have been shown to be more effective at treating osteoarthritis.

Frankincense essential oil is used by many people with rheumatoidarthritis for rain relief. Despite the fact that Frankincense cannot be used to treat RA, it is an important part of rain management. It has been shown in various studies to reduce inflammation, rain, and stiffness. Frankincense has been shown to have positive immune system effects in laboratory studies.

Pycnogenol (Maritime Bark) is a very effective herb for reducing vascular inflammation, healing injuries, and treating ulcers. It has been discovered to be one of the most potent anti-inflammatory herbs. According to studies, rycnogenol can neutralize free radicals 50 to 100 times more effectively than vitamin E. It lowers the risk of blood loss and clotting.

It can be used to treat allergies and asthma, as well as high blood pressure, osteoarthritis (OA), diabetes, endometriosis (ED), attention deficit hyperactivity disorder (ADHD), and retinorathy, an eye condition.

Rcynogenol is a supplement that can help rostmenorexic women with their symptoms. The anti-oxidant effects of rycnogenol on the endothelium led to this conclusion. It's the thin membrane that lines the insides of our blood vessels and our hearts. The same study discovered that rycnogenol increases the availability of nitric oxide, which aids in circulation.

In another study, rcynogenol was found to reduce the amount of rain and swelling in patients with chronic vein insufficiency. This occurs when the blood vessels in the legs have trouble returning blood to the heart.

In a 2009 study of diabetic retinopathy and diabetes in its early stages, 18 of 24 patients had improved vision. The rlacebo had no effect on the participants' vision.

It's an anti-inflammatory that can help you avoid strokes and heart attacks. It's used to treat varicose veins and other "anti-aging" products. Maritime Bark Carules can be purchased online or at your local health food store.

THE LIFESTYLE APPROACH, CHAPTER 7

We want to be able to enjoy our newfound health and the way our bodies and minds feel after removing the toxic substances we've been consuming through poor diets. There are numerous strategies available to assist you in achieving this new way of life.

Let's take a closer look at a few of them.

TURNING TECHNOLOGY OFF

Technology is everywhere in this day and age. It was designed to bring people together in the first place. It was explained to us that a simple email, text message, phone call, or video could allow people to connect, communicate, inform, and form relationships. For many of us, it appears to work the other way around.

Our world is filled with a sense of impermanence and a surplus of emrtiness. How can we make our lives more fulfilling? These are some ideas and suggestions to help you return to a state of calm, calm, clear thinking, and availability to yourself and others.

The average person touches their screens 261 times per day, according to studies. This appears to be quite a lot. Let's just say we're one of those people, even if we don't think we are. We all know we're rhone-obsessed. Others constantly interrupt us with information, and we constantly check texts, emails, and the news. We also use the Internet to check the weather, order food, get directions, and play rlaying games. Being available for others 24 hours a day, seven days a week is extremely stressful.

It has been established that technology, particularly Smartphones, is addictive. Every time we open a text, email, or social media site, or even check the air quality on our phones, we release endorphins. Endorphins are the hormones responsible for our "Feel Goods." It works in the same way that alcohol, marijuana, and other mood-altering substances do.

People who are exposed to blue light from screens are at risk for a condition known as "Computer Face." Premature wrinkles, frown lines, jowls, furrowed foreheads, and a Turkey neck characterize that face.' 'Screen dermatitis' is another term for it. Eye strain is also caused by too much time spent in front of a screen.

Facebook and other social media sites are contributing to what researchers refer to as "Fear of Missing Out" (FOMO for short). Not everyone has access to all of the wonderful activities, amazing vacations, birthday greetings, and gatherings with friends and family that are broadcast on social media. People may feel excluded and even inadequate as a result of their experiences. FOMO affects young women and girls in particular. It creates a mental environment conducive to loneliness and depression, regardless of age or gender.

Of course, technology isn't all bad. It's how we use it that keeps us from living a fuller life.

So, what's a person to do?

First and foremost, we must accept that real life is right in front of us. There are some moments and experiences in life that will never be duplicated. This day's sunrise or sunset will never happen again. We'll miss those conversations with people we care about if we're glued to our phones. When we look away from our screens and think we're ready to interact, our children, pets, and significant others may not be present. When we consider cutting back on technology, this should be our driving force.

Let's begin with mobile phones. Set aside "Phone Free Time" during mealtimes. This will assist us in connecting with others.

both to others and to ourselves Taking calls during mealtimes was once considered impolite. With the widespread use of cellphones, this appears to have loosened considerably. What's more, guess what. Even so, it's still impolite. There are some professions that require people to be available 24 hours a day, at least on scheduled days. This isn't the case. When the meal isn't being served, phones should be turned off. For many of us, even turning off notifications but leaving it in front of us is still a temptation. Remove it from the room.

Make "coffee breaks" on your phone. Take a break for even 15 minutes a couple of times a day. But don't count on yourself to be self-disciplined. Set your phone to notify you of your break times, which may sound ironic. Then put it somewhere where it won't be accessible for that period of time.

If you have to check your phone at a traffic light, put it in the backseat or even the trunk. Instead, put on some music. If you have a passenger, speak with them. Your passenger, as well as all other drivers on the road, will thank you, whether you can hear them or not. Getting directions on our phones has become fairly commonplace in recent years. If at all possible, hand the phone to a passenger who can tell you which turn to take next.

Notify others of your new limitations. Tell them when it's okay for them to try to contact you or when you'll be able to respond. You'll have to apologize if you don't. You'll be forced to return to your screen, and you'll lose control of your free time as a result.

Consumption is closely linked to screen time. You'll probably find that limiting your screen time helps you spend less money on things you don't really need. Instead, use that money to have fun with the people you care about. Spend some money and time on a getaway for yourself to relax and recover from the stresses of life. It isn't necessary to go all out.

WALKING

In chapter 5, we talked about yoga as an approach to strengthen your body, to improve energy and vitality and achieve some peace and tranquility in this hectic world.

Walking is another type of exercise that can help with social, emotional, and physical strength. Walking supports many aspects of a healthy lifestyle. Walking is easier on the joints and heart than running or jogging. Walking is now being hailed as "the closest thing we have to a wonder drug" according to former director of Centers for Disease Control and Prevention, Dr. Thomas Frieden. Many positive gains from this form of exercise are available to most. Even starting out with a small walk can evolve into much looked forward to regimen. Let's look at some of the things walking can do for you.

OXYGEN AND CIRCULATION

As you walk, the improved circulation supplies the brain with the required oxygen and glucose for optimum functioning. You can even become a little smarter by walking! By bringing up the heart rate and lowering blood pressure, you are protecting both your heart and brain. University of Colorado at Boulder and the University of Tennessee found in their studies that post- menopausal women were able to lower their blood pressure by n points in 6 months. Thirty minutes of walking a day were linked to a 20 percent less risk of stroke in a similar study group, and by stepping up the pace, risk of stroke was reduced by 40 percent.

STAYING HYDRATED

The human body is 60 percent water. Staying hydrated after exercise and through-out the day only makes sense to maintain maximum function of our brains, the heart, the transportation of nutrients to cells and to flush out toxins.

Weight Loss -Staying hydrated assists with weight loss. The results of several studies reported in the journalObesityshowed that more weight was lost by those who regularly drank the recommended amount of water than those who did not.

Cardiovascular Health Drinking water lowers the risk of heart attacks. When dehydrated, arteries become narrow. If there is cholesterol and plaque being stored within these arteries, the risk of heart attacks becomes very high. Keeping hydrated improves the way arteries function.

Flushing Toxins The elimination of waste is hindered by being dehydrated. The kidneys and colon rely on being hydrated in order to function properly. Being hydrated prevents the occurrence of kidney stones. Proper hydration protects against rheumatoid arthritis and eases the pain of osteoarthritis.

Boosts Energy Levels The Journal of Athletic Training and Nutrition published findings that staying hydrated before, during and after exercising not only lessened fatigue, but also boosted endurance.

Avoid the single -use plastic water bottles. Besides polluting the environment with discarded plastic, drinking out of these bottles isn't good for us. Plastic bottles contain bisphenol A (BPA), a chemical used to make the plastic clear and durable. It's an endocrine disruptor and has been linked to neurological issues, cancer, and early puberty in young girls among other problems.

BPA has been found in growing fetuses and placentas.

Also found in the plastic of water bottles and other food storage containers is another chemical called phthalates, which is another endocrine disruptor.

Presently, the FDA doesn't regulate phthalates as it is found in trace amounts in plastic. But when you consider the frequency that plastic is used as a container, it really is prevalent in our lives.

Utilize metal water bottles to keep the hydration process safe. They can be washed again and again. The purity of the water from plastic has been debated over the past few years. It's typically only as clean as tap water.

Be good to yourself. Stay hydrated. Choose a method that will match an anti-inflammatory lifestyle.

WALKING BOOSTS IMMUNITY

Walking counteracts the effects of weight -producing genetics. Researchers at Harvard examined 32 weight producing genes to evaluate how they contribute to body weight. Over 12,000 people were part of the study. It was discovered that those who walked briskly every day for an hour the effect of these genes was cut by 50 percent.

Researchers agree that any sort of exercise helps prevent certain types of cancer. Walking actually prevents the formation of breast cancer. The American Cancer Society conducted a study of women who walked at least 7 hours per week. It was discovered that these women had a 14 percent reduced risk of developing breast cancer compared to women who only walked 3-4 hours per week.

Just by walking 30 minutes a day, your immune cells are strengthened with oxygen improving the function of B-cells, T-cells and releases clumps of WBCs (white blood cells) found in the renal system and urinary tract. A study of 1,000 men and women reported that during the cold and flu season walkers had a 43 percent lower chance of getting sick. By walking only 20 minutes a day for at least 5 days a week, the test group experienced fewer symptoms and a shorter duration of colds and flu, if they became sick at all.

WALKING STRENGTHENS BONES

The gentle strike of your feet against the sidewalk, ground or track squeezes the cartilage sending oxygen and nutrients to your joints. Walking produces vitamin D, which nourishes bones. You'll experience a reduction in joint pain because of this nutritious lubrication and makes

the threat of osteoarthritis less likely. This is really important to arthritis sufferers. Muscles around the joints are strengthened. Studies have shown that 5 miles a week can ward off the development of arthritis in the first place.

SLOWS MENTAL DECLINE

A study of 6,000 women, age 65 plus at the University of California, San Francisco found that there was a significant decline in age-related memory issues. From walking 2.5 miles per day, there was a 17 percent decline in memory as opposed to those women who only walked a half mile per day. The second group suffered declines at 25 percent.

Walking reduces the risk of Alzheimer's. The group of men ages of 71 to 93 studied at the University of Virginia Health System in Charlottesville, had half the incidence of Alzheimer's disease if they walked more than a quarter of a mile a day than those men who walked less.

If you walk regularly at a moderate pace, a pace wherein you can still hold a conversation, your risk of Alzheimer's and impaired memory is largely decreased.

LONGER LIVES People who regularly exercise by walking in their fifties and sixties are 35 percent more likely to live longer than those who do not walk. A Harvard study of 17,000 graduates showed that they lived longer than their sedentary peers. A study by the American Geriatrics Society determined that people between the ages of 70 to 90 who maintained some sort of physical activity lived longer than their counterparts.

It appears that all forms of inflammatory diseases can improve with regular walking. A more recent study from Arthritis and Therapy suggested that interval walking improves the immune function in people with rheumatoid arthritis. David Nieman, professor of public health at Appalachian State University, as well as being the director of the Human Performance Lab there, has spent nine years studying the effects of exercise on the immune system. He said, "We found that, after three hours of exercise, these immune cells retreat back to the tissues they came from." This means that when immune cells come across destructive pathogens, they are able to destroy them.

You may have heard of Blue Zones. These are parts of the world where people live longer than the average. The term "Blue Zones"was trademarked by Dan Buettner in November of 2005 in an article he wrote for the National Geographic. The article was about the lifestyles of the long- lived residents in Okinawa, Japan, Sardinia, the Nicoya Peninsula in Costa Rica, and Loma Linda, California. Aside from eating an antiinflammatory diet or a Mediterranean diet, all of these people are physically active. All include walking as part of their fitness routines.

Walking offers the opportunity to connect with others. Your neighbors, your friends and family members would probably enjoy the chance to socialize and establish a routine for exercise. Look into walking clubs. There are opportunities to support various social causes through organized walks.

This is a great way to broaden your support system and build a new circle of friends.

Overall, walking and exercise are important to add to your new approach to health. It supports your immune system that can then more effectively fight the inflammatory response that your body has been dealing with. The results will be profound. Walking reduces stress. Your mood will improve. From the extra activity and oxygen intake, you'll sleep better at night. Digestion improves. Walking fights the effects of weight producing hormones. It even reduces the risk for type 2 diabetes. Exercise and walking are important. Invest in this time.

MEDITATION

Anxiety and chronic stress trigger inflammation. To deal with uncomfortable feelings, the body sends inflammation markers to help cope with the experience. These markers release the stress hormone cortisol. Cortisol generates the harmful inflammation producing chemical, cytokine, that wreaks havoc on a person's immune system. The reaction to stress can lead to depression, sleepless nights, anxiety, over-eating, high blood pressure, and possibly turning to substances that appear to help us escape challenging realities. All of these are negative coping behaviors and reactions that are harmful to our health.

It is imperative, then, to learn how to cope with stress. We can't escape stress. It arrives to us in all kinds of forms. Good stress with a new job, a new baby, a move can still be challenging. And, of course, there is the bad stress.

Thousands of studies on meditation have shown that it benefits mental and physical health. These studies consistently show that diseases are managed better and even disappear, sleep is improved, stress is reduced, focus is improved, various addictions are better managed, pain management is controlled, and even relationships get better when meditation is practiced.

A study of over 2,400 individuals using mindful meditation showed a reduction in anxiety among those who suffered from a variety of mental health issues such as social anxiety, panic disorders, obsessive-compulsive disorders, and job-related anxiety. Another study of 4,600 subjects found long-term ease from depression.

A practice called "Mindful Meditation" has been proven to reduce the inflammatory response created by stress. One study showed that this type of meditation reduced the inflammatory response in 1,300 individuals. The people with the highest levels of stress were found to experience the greatest benefit.

Harvard has concurred with what yogis have been saying for thousands of years that with meditation we increase our emotional capacity for happiness, empathy, better moods, creativity, and viewing problems as smaller and more manageable.

The Journal of Biobehavioral Medicine published findings of a study of brain alterations consistent with mindful meditation practices. Over an 8week clinical trial in a workplace setting that evaluated emotions of healthy employees, the findings from brain electrical activity were consistent with reports of increased positive emotions.

Meditation is strongly liked to improvements in physical health. Harvard's studies on meditation confirm that there are reductions in tension related pain such as pain associated with ulcers, muscle and joint pain, tension headaches and ulcers. A Wake Forest study on meditation confirmed in 20iithat after only 4 days of mindful meditation their subjects experienced a reduction in pain by 57 percent and pain intensity was reduced by lessened by 40 percent.

The Mayo Clinic has released research findings that back up meditation's capacity to help people relax.

asthma, cancer, chronic pain syndromes, heart disease, high blood pressure, and irritable bowel syndrome are just a few of the disorders that may be managed. These are the results from October of 2017.

There are many different meditation methods and practices to choose from. There will undoubtedly be one that appeals to you among the various sorts available.

Progressive Meditation or Body Scan

Block out at least 20 to 30 minutes of time when you won't be disturbed to complete a body scan or progressive meditation. Find a spot where you can be alone and not troubled by other people's wants or responsibilities hanging over your head. This is a chance to get away from it all.

As you begin, pay attention to the portions of your body that make touch with the chair or mat you're sitting on. Take a few moments to ensure that you are as comfortable as you possibly can. Even a little alteration may have a significant impact on your capacity to relax and let go of tension in your body.

Consider yourself on a tour of your own body. Begin by noting how the clothing you're wearing feel. Take note of the texture and weight of any blankets that may be draped over you.

Make your way to your various bodily components. Don't try to envision your bodily parts; instead, feel them. Simply sense them. Concentrate on the feelings on the top of your head, including your forehead, ears, eyebrows, eyes, cheeks, and lips. Just start at the top and work your way down. You may also start at your toes and work your way up. Pay attention to the feelings in the soles of your feet, ankles, calves, knees, thighs, and other areas. Allow a body part to fade out of your consciousness after scanning it.

You'll probably be instructed to link body parts if you have an instructor or are utilizing an app. Then you'll join your head to your neck. After that, join your neck to your torso. Finally, you'll notice how your skin wraps around your body.

Body scans come in a variety of shapes and sizes. This is a straightforward description of how things work. People with chronic pain conditions benefit from body scans. It allows them to see that their pain does not extend throughout their entire body. They may find that some regions of their bodies are pain-free.

Yoga Nidra is a meditative state in which

"Sleep with awareness" is the meaning of yoga nidra. It's a relaxing technique that aims to relieve mental, emotional, and bodily tension. Some people say that a session of yoga nidra is as restorative as sleeping for several hours.

Meditation and yoga nidra are not the same thing. Meditation is usually done while sitting. You're relaxed, aware, and comfortable. You are laying down while you perform yoga nidra.

One anchor is usually used in meditation to keep your attention focused. It's usually the breath that causes the problem. You are led during a yoga nidra session. Step by step, your attention is drawn to certain locations.

Yoga nidra allows you to enter a profound stage of conscious slumber. You're not in a waking state of awareness, and you've passed through the dreaming stage. You're awake, yet you're in a deep slumber.

The advantages of yoga nidra include, but are not limited to, insomnia relief, anxiety reduction, PTSD management, and chronic pain management. It aids in the recovery of those who have been stressed. Yoga nidra aids in the recovery of those who are unwell. It may aid in the treatment of drug dependence.

In today's fast-paced, high-tech society, the necessity for this relaxing exercise is becoming more apparent. These are the most recent data on sleep deprivation in the United States.

- Sleep deprivation affects more than 30% of the general population -Insomnia affects more than 60% of the over 60 population -More than 50% of Americans lose sleep due to worry and stress -

More than 10% of Americans use prescription sleeping pills, with many more using over-the-counter sleep aids.

As we all know, stress and lack of sleep induce inflammation, which leads to a variety of ailments and disorders. Mental health concerns are one of them, and they may cause inflammation in the physical body. Yoga nidra is a kind of meditation that may help you unwind from the stresses of contemporary life while also providing a restful night's sleep.

Meditation for Mindfulness

This is the visual representation of mindfulness meditation. People sit with their hands resting on their knees, their feet flat on the floor, and their eyes closed. They're sitting in a peaceful area that they've made for themselves. They are taught to concentrate on the present moment by observing physiological sensations, thoughts, and emotions. The breath is given special care.

Mindfulness meditation practitioners claim to think more clearly and have less stress in their life.

"Our brains wander all the time, either analyzing the past or preparing for the future," says Suzanne Westbrook, a Harvard internal medicine specialist who just retired.

By observing when your mind wanders, mindfulness teaches you how to pay attention in the present moment. Return your attention to your breathing. It's a location where we can unwind and calm down." She mentioned this while conducting an eight-week stress-reduction course.

Because of the inflammation caused by stress, we are at a significantly greater risk of stroke, heart disease, and a variety of other ailments when we can't relax our bodies and quiet our thoughts. Continuous stress causes our bodies to create cortisol, which is responsible for a variety of ailments, including these.

The goal of mindfulness meditation isn't to change ourselves from who we are now. Its goal is to educate us how to be completely present and accepting of whatever is going on in our lives at the time. Acceptance allows us to let go more easily, according to mindfulness meditation. We won't be conflicted in our heads about things we can't control in the first place. This helps to relieve tension.

The concept claims that when we strive to avoid suffering by clinging to pleasure, the reverse happens. Our enjoyment is not sustained by our attempts to escape and dominate. We suffer as a result of it.

We can show up for our life when we are conscious. We aren't living our lives longing for something different. We won't be able to live fully and be present if we're worried about whether or not something nice will endure.

Body, breath, and ideas are the three main components of the practice.

Create your surroundings first. It might be as easy as lighting a candle or burning incense for many folks. This serves as a reminder of life's impermanence. Others make it more personal by adorning altars with flowers, photos, and artifacts from their own culture.

Take a seat on a cushion or a chair. Check to see whether you'll be able to sit up straight. Avoid selecting a chair that you know will cause back pain. Place your hands on your thighs and lower your head. Your eyes are gentle and rest on the ground.

When your mind wanders, don't resist it. It will stray. The goal is to return your attention back to your breath, body, and the surroundings you've established.

Breathing is the second phase of the exercise. Just take a deep breath. There isn't any unique method used. What's intended to happen is that you pay attention to how you're feeling right now. Don't stress about managing or regulating your breath. Allowing yourself to get engrossed in what you're doing with your breathing is a bad idea.

Working with your ideas is the last step in the exercise. People's thoughts stray. We're thinking about the past and what's going on this afternoon. We'll indulge in a few fantasies. We may recall a beloved music from a long time ago. Thoughts might become confused and overlapping. When this occurs, softly, very slowly return your attention to your breathing. Don't be too hard on yourself. This occurs often, particularly when you're just starting out with this kind of meditation. It is not the goal of this meditation to make us stop thinking. The purpose of most meditations isn't to become completely blank. It isn't even close to becoming a component of a focused meditation practice. If you're new to meditation, start with meditating for 10 minutes. You'll gradually increase your time to 20 to 30 minutes. A 45-minute meditation will be a pleasant habit if you've been doing this for a while. There is no expectation that you meditate for a certain amount of time. Acceptance is the theme of this meditation.

Meditation in the Zen style

Zen meditation, also referred to as Zazen, is a Buddhist-inspired meditation technique.

Lotus position (sitting on a mat with legs crossed) is a common starting point for practitioners. The emphasis is on the inside of the body. Some claim that counting breaths does this, while others claim that no counting is required.

Zen meditation emphasizes mental awareness. The practitioner's eyes are slightly open while doing Zen meditation. They gently steer away from any thoughts in their heads, attempting to think about nothing at all. The idea is to tap into the unconscious mind after practitioners have learned to restrict their thoughts from straying. You'll be more aware of preconceived notions and have a better understanding of yourself once you've mastered this.

Mediation on Loving Kindness

This is dubbed a "radical act of love" by some. As the pace of contemporary life continues to increase, causing stress and instability, an increasing number of individuals are turning to this sort of meditation for self-care.

One of the most effective antidotes to the anxiety and wrath of our current social experience may be loving kindness meditation. This practice is a non-judgmental and non-reactive way of dealing with the anxiety-inducing realities of our current society, which are so inflammatory to our minds and bodies.

What's the deal here? Take a seat in a position that is convenient for you. You can sit or lie down. Choose the best position for you. Allow yourself to relax and be present by focusing on your breathing. Allow yourself to get carried away.

After that, visualize someone you love or someone who loves you. Allow yourself to be carried away by the feelings that this relationship has brought up in you. Tap into the emotions and sentiments that this individual has bestowed onto you. Take a few deep breaths and allow yourself to get carried away by your emotions. Bathe in the knowledge that this person or these people accept and love you exactly as you are.

You may believe that you are unworthy of such intense love. It's irrelevant. It does not matter. It doesn't matter what you look like; what matters is that you're appreciated for who you are. You are not who you once were or might have been. Allow yourself to be enveloped in the feelings of love.

When you're ready, try becoming both the source and the recipient of these emotions. Make these sentiments your own so you may share them with others. Keep a close eye on your pulse. Relax and take in these sentiments of unconditional love, forgiveness, and self-acceptance.

You might say a mantra to yourself while you relax in this zone of self-love and compassion. They should be expressed in the present tense, as though the events are now taking place. Something along the lines of: "I am secure." I'm in a good mood and satisfied with my life. I've recovered my health and am no longer sick. At least three times, repeat one or two similar statements. When you first start this portion of the exercise, you may feel a bit silly, but after a while, you'll realize it's a part of how you actually feel about yourself. During this exercise, it is common for your thoughts to wander. Remember, this isn't about evaluating yourself. Allow yourself to return to love and compassion sentiments. Self-compassion is key.

Many individuals wonder, "Why am I focused so much on myself?" after learning about this technique. "It feels like you're focusing on yourself." This meditation's objective is to help us identify and experience our place in the universe. We are neither superior nor inferior to others. We belong, and we must include ourselves in this loving practice in order to honestly and unconditionally give our love and acceptance with others.

Loving kindness is a kind of energy field that can extend out to everyone, but it must start with yourself.

ourselves. It may be extended to persons with whom you've had a squabble, as well as those who have been rude to you. It's a story about forgiveness and love.

The anti-inflammatory lifestyle is based on long-established methods that will lead us in the future. Experiment with various meditation techniques to see what works best for you. Styles may be changed as necessary. Remember that there is no one-size-fits-all approach to meditation. Meditation's goal is to alleviate tension, quiet your mind, and make your mind and emotions more at peace.

GRATITUDE IN THE WORKSHOP

Gratitude improves cortisol levels by altering our stress response. Inflammation is exacerbated by high cortisol levels, which must be reduced or eliminated. Gratitude allows us to see things from different perspectives. Anxiety is managed in response to events that are beyond our control. Gratitude helps us break free from worry cycles that can harm our health in the long run.

Gratitude strengthens relationships, makes people happier, and improves health, according to studies on the subject. It boosts your stress-resistance. Hormones are balanced by gratitude. According to research, cultivating gratitude promotes positive hormonal changes while lowering cortisol levels, which is a stress hormone.

On a biochemical level, gratitude feels good. When you have an emotional connection to the things you are grateful for, the frontal lobe of your brain is activated. Dopamine and serotonin hormones are released, resulting in feelings of awe and comfort.

Gratitude can help you feel less hungry. We don't feel a lack of abundance when we're truly grateful. There isn't any more that we require. More food, fun, activity, and material possessions are not required. Cravings are reduced, allowing us to appreciate the people we care about, the things we own, the food we eat, and the health benefits that these foods provide.

Make it a habit to get the most out of this technique. At the start of the day, some people enjoy thinking about what they are grateful for. Others use it to wind down before going to sleep. Think of two or three things for which you are grateful, and spend time visualizing and reaching for the emotion that person or thing provides. By focusing on the emotions you experience as you practice thankfulness, gratitude enhances the mind-body connection. The center of energy in your body is your heart. You can widen your range of experiences and emotions by practicing gratitude.

Keeping a gratitude journal is a great way to keep track of your accomplishments. As you review lists or written thoughts about what makes you thankful, just looking at it can bring a sense of calm to you. It should be kept in a convenient location. It can be placed on a table next to a favorite chair or by your bedside. It's more likely that you'll pick it up and use it if it's visible.

It is not required that new items be added to the journal on a daily basis. It's fine to say "thank you" as many times as you want, as long as your gratitude is genuine. You can express your gratitude for that daughter, son, significant other, parent, job, or pet on a number of occasions. Perhaps you're relieved that your vehicle hasn't broken down. You might be grateful for the garden you helped to plant. You can be thankful for clean water and air, as well as electricity and a roof over your head. There's no end to the list. It's possible that one of your entry items is about you. Don't forget about yourself! Don't take yourself for granted. Consider all of your achievements, big and small.

Allow yourself to bask in the glory of your achievements. It's your due.

It is easier to stay in the present if we concentrate on what we currently have. This isn't the case.

Worrying about what we had or might have in the future. Right now, we're standing here. The way we see life changes when we are present. We enjoy things more when we're present. We have the option of slowing down and savoring our food. We take in the view of the sky and trees. We can smell the breezes and appreciate the flower scents. We've discovered that we're paying more attention. Those who are important to us can be seen clearly.

Gratitude is an endearing quality that spreads quickly. You'll say "thank you" more frequently and with genuine gratitude. You might notice that you're attracting more friends after some time. And they'll most likely share your values.

GET OUT OF THE CITY AND INTO THE WOODS.

Everyone used to spend more time in nature than they do now, even just a generation or two ago. As a result, in both big cities and small towns, people are more stressed and anxious. Psychologists have recently published research indicating that mental health disorders like depression and anxiety are on the rise. We've discussed how meditation can lower inflammation by improving mood and calming nerves. However, we haven't yet discussed how returning to nature can help us relax.

Gary Bratman, a graduate student, has been researching the psychological differences between people who live in cities and those who spend time in natural settings. In a study he and his colleagues conducted while at Stanford University's Emmett Interdisciplinary Program in Environment and Resources, they discovered that volunteers who walked through the lush campus were happier and more alert than volunteers who walked through heavy multi-lane traffic for the same amount of time. Mr. Bratman and his colleagues reported on the levels of brain activity in the subgenual prefrontal cortex of all volunteers in Proceedings of the National Academy of Sciences. Unsurprisingly, test subjects who walked around the lush, green campus improved their mental health. Brain activity was found to be less agitated in the study. They were happier because they didn't spend as much time brooding. The findings "strongly suggest that getting out into natural environments" could be an easy and effective way for people living in cities to relax and improve their moods, according to the researchers.

Some of you may believe that a scientific study isn't required to obtain the same outcomes. The majority of us find that spending time in nature, whether it's in the mountains, by a lake, or by the sea, improves our well-being. We wonder why we don't spend more time with "Mother Nature," because it benefits us so much.

Our mood and attitude improve as a result of this. Our memories have become sharper as a result of this. The feeling of being alone is lessened. Our nerves are calmed by the forest's scents. Aromatherapy, in a nutshell! After spending time outdoors, we sleep better. We have a better quality of life when we are outside.

Walking in the Natural Environment

There is more information about the advantages of taking a nature walk than there has ever been before. There is an increasing body of research on the mental and physical benefits of walking in nature. Recent studies have even shown that taking a "short micro-break" by looking at a natural scene can help test subjects relax. These rejuvenating moments have been shown to have a positive effect on the adult brain, leading to longer attention spans. It also allows kids to perform better on cognitive tests.

Reduced stress, improved cardio-vascular health, healthy weight, stronger bones and cartilage, improved self-esteem and mood, and increased creative thinking have all been discovered in recent studies. Walking outdoors makes people happier than working out in a gym.

The cellular activity that's been associated with nature walks through forests in particular have indicated possible links to production of anticancer proteins. The levels of these proteins have been found to last up to 7 days after a stroll through the forest. Studies from Japan, have discovered that in regions with large areas of forest that there are lower mortality rates from cancer even after considering cigarette smoking and lower socioeconomic status of the test subjects.

Nature walks have been proven to lower blood pressure. Research has confirmed that there is weight loss associated with walking outside. Nature walks help stave off colds and flu. It's been proven that our brains work better. The vitamin D we get from being outside and in sunlight reduces inflammation. Time in nature can improve longevity.

In children it's been demonstrated that spending time outdoors can protect their eyesight. The risk of developing nearsightedness (myopia) is greatly reduced. A 2012 review of this research concurred with those findings.

The objective of taking a nature walk doesn't have to be anything more than taking a break and enjoying the outdoors. However, there are a lot of things you can do to enhance the experience when the walk feels like it's becoming a little too routine. Here are some before, during and after activities that might bring the experience into a sharper focus.

- Focus in on the five senses. Pay marked attention to what you see, what you feel, what you taste, what you hear and smell and describe these things to yourself or your walking partner.

-

Walk at different times of the day or evening. You might notice things that you hadn't before during your regular walking time.

-Sketch a picture of what you see. Skip taking pictures and selfies.

-

Lay on a blanket and look up into the trees or the sky. Make cloud "pictures."

-Go barefoot and feel the grass, the dirt, the sand, and the water on your

feet.-Catch fireflies in the evening and let them go. It might bring back a lovely childhood memory.

- Collect fall leaves. Use them for a project at home.

-Paint rocks you find. Make people and houses or things you saw on your walk.

-Keep a journal about your walks.

-Listen to the birds, the air, the water.

John Muir said, "In ever walk with Nature, one receives far more than he seeks." We all know this to be true. Nature walks are lovely opportunities for making discoveries, being creative, for getting relaxed, and just to enjoy ourselves. Taking the time to give ourselves this gift is a treasure.

CHAPTER 8:TWO WEEK DIET PLAN

The anti -inflammatory diet should contain pre-biotics, omega-gs, fiber, protein, healthy fats, vitamins, minerals and anti-oxidants. The meals should include whole grains, fatty fish, legumes, fresh fruit and vegetables. Remember to drink eight 8-ounces glasses of water daily, and only a moderate amount of red wine if allowed by your doctor. Keep in mind that it's a plant- based diet, with little or no red meat. Here is a place to start to get into the habit to cook foods that will feed your body and reduce your inflammation. The following meal plan ideas require little preparation and can be altered for convenience.

Week 1

Breakfast Choices:\s-Oatmeal with berries and Greek Yogurt\s-Raspberry/Strawberry/Blueberry Smoothie\s-Buckwheat Pancakes with Berries)

-Granola, with Berries and Greek Yogurt

-Quinoa with Riced Cauliflower and Cinnamon

-Poached Salmon, Avocado and Poached Egg on Multi-grain Toast Muesli with Raspberries and Greek Yogurt

Lunch Choices:\s-Avocado, Hummus and Radish Sandwich on Sprouted Bread\s-Crushed Kale Salad, Red Onions and Mushrooms with Multi-grain Bread*

-Lemon/Garlic Zoodies and Green Salad

-Black Eyed Peas with Beets and Hazelnut Salad and Pita Bread*

-Color Bowl Salad Made with Vegetables with Color and Quinoa

-Stir Fried Tofu with Broccoli and Shredded Carrot -Roasted Root Vegetables, Quinoa and Feta Salad

Dinner Choices:\s-Curried Potatoes with Egg

-Salmon Cakes with Dark, Green Vegetable and Tomato Juice

-Vegetarian Chili

-Chicken Breast with Sweet Potatoes and Spinach and Basil Salad Pan

Fried Trout, Broccoli and Quinoa, Small Glass of Red Wine -Lentil and Chicken Soup with Sweet Potato and Spinach* Walnut Crusted Baked Salmon, Black Rice, Balsamic and Parmesan Brussels Sprouts*

Snack Choices:\s-Tart, red cherries

-Handful of Almonds with a Small Cup of Cantaloupe

-Plain Greek Yogurt with Berries\s-Cottage Cheese with Walnuts and Cinnamon\s-Sliced Tomato with Olives\s-Small Handful of Dark Chocolate Chips and Walnuts

Week 2: Breakfast Choices: "Scrambled Eggs with Turmeric and Multigrain Toast "Whole Grain English Muffin Topped with Ricotta, Almonds and Honey

"Oatmeal with Cinnamon, Dates, Honey and Greek Yogurt* "Two Slices of Whole Grain Toast with Ricotta Cheese and Chopped

Berries "Baked Eggs with Avocado and Feta Cheese* "Whole Wheat Pancakes Topped with Ricotta and Berries "

Pan Fried Egg with Multi-grain Toast, Tomatoes and Avocados

Lunch Choices: "Grilled Eggplant, Zucchini and Onion on Whole Wheat Toast "Egg Frittata with Asparagus and Green Tossed Salad "Mixed Salad Greens with Olives and Cherry Tomatoes "Roasted Spicy Anchovies with Avocados, Sprouts on Multi-grain Toast "Bell Peppers, Olives, Sun-dried Tomatoes and Spinach on Quinoa* "Roasted Vegetables in Pita Pockets with Hummus "

White Bean Soup with Chicken, Raw Vegetable Slices

Dinner Choices: "Arugula and Spinach Salad with Zucchini, Cherry Tomatoes, Boiled Egg

and Sprouts with Pita Pocket and Hummus -Whole Grain Pasta with Sun-dried Tomatoes, Grilled Vegetables and Rosemary, Small Glass of Red Wine

"Grilled Trout, Baked Sweet Potato and Green Salad "Zoodle Spaghetti with Basil Pesto and Sliced Tomatoes

"Pita Pocket Topped with Feta, Steamed Spinach, Sun -dried Tomatoes and Kalamata Olives "

Grilled Tuna Steak with Baked Potato and Chives -Roast Chicken with Turmeric, Wild Rice and Mint, Tossed Green Salad*

Snack Choices: "Two Plums and Almonds "Handful of Dried Fruit "Red Grapes and Walnuts "Hard Cheese and Strawberries "Plain Greek Yogurt with Drizzle of Honey "Red Bell Pepper with Guacamole, Small Glass of Red Wine "Apple Slices with Peanut Butter

RECIPES BREAKFAST: Poached Salmon, Avocado and Poached Egg on Multi -grain Toast Ingredients:

1/2 C. dry white wine 1/2 C. water

2 lbs. salmon filets cut into 4 pieces 4 eggs

1T. extra virgin olive oil 1/4 tsp. freshly grated garlic 1 tsp. dried parsley

2 avocados sliced Basil leaves

6 slices of multi-grain toast Sea salt and pepper to taste

Bring the wine and water to a boil in a large pan. Add the salmon and spices into the wine and water, reduce heat to a simmer on medium heat. The salmon should be firm but tender after 10 minutes.

To poach the eggs, bring water to a simmer on medium heat in a medium-sized pan. Crack eggs, one by one, into the water and cook for 2 minutes. Remove the pan from the heat and let it sit for 8-10 minutes.

With a slotted spoon, lift eggs out of the water and let drain on a towel for a couple of minutes. On each slice of warm multi-grain toast, place the salmon, the basil leaves and an egg on top. Garnish with avocado slices.

Selves 4. Oatmeal with Cinnamon, Dates, Honey and Greek Yogurt Ingredients:

1 C. Traditional breakfast oats 1/4 C. dates

Honey and cinnamon to taste

1/2 C. Greek yogurt for each serving

Bring 1 3/4 C. water to a boil. Add the oats and stir for 1 minute as water continues to boil. Remove from heat, cover and let water absorb for 10 minutes.

Serve with dates, honey and cinnamon to taste with 1/2 C. Greek yogurt. Serves 2. Baked Eggs with Avocado and Feta Cheese Ingredients:

3 T. extra virgin olive oil 1 small red onion chopped

1 clove garlic finely minced

1/2 jalapeno pepper finely minced, with seeds discarded 1T. oregano

1 tsp. chili pepper 1 tsp. paprika Fresh basil leaves

Sea salt and pepper to taste 6 eggs

1 avocado sliced 1/2 C. feta cheese

Preheat oven to 400 degrees F.

In a large cast iron skillet or other heavy cookware, saute the small red onion, the jalapeno and garlic in olive oil until the onion just begins to turn brown. Add spices and continue to saute for another 2 minutes.

Crack eggs into the onion mixture that has been spread evenly in the pan. If you don't have cast iron, you can transfer the mixture into a 9 x 13" pan that has been prepped with a light coating of olive oil.

Bake for 15-18 minutes. Garnish with avocado slices and basil leaves. Serves 4 to 6.

LUNCH: Crushed Kale Salad, Red Onions and Mushrooms with Multi-grain Bread Ingredients:

1 bunch kale

1 medium red onion sliced 3/4 lb. sliced white mushrooms

Dressing: 1/4 C. balsamic vinegar 1/2 C. extra virgin olive oil 1/2 tsp. thyme

Saute red onions in 2 T. extra virgin olive oil on medium heat. In another pan, saute mushrooms in 2 T. extra virgin olive oil on medium heat, as well.

Rinse and dry kale. Crush in your hands before tearing (it makes it sweeter). Combine the onion, the mushrooms and kale and toss. Top with dressing.

Dressing: Combine the balsamic vinegar, the oil and the thyme and stir or shake.

Selves 4. Bell Peppers, Olives, Sun-dried Tomatoes and Spinach on Quinoa Ingredients:

1 bell pepper sliced

1/2 C. sliced Kalamata olives

1/2 C. sundried tomatoes 2 C. fresh spinach

2 C. cooked quinoa

2 T. extra virgin olive oil

Prepare quinoa as directed on package. Rinse and dry spinach. Saute the sliced bell pepper in olive oil until tender and add olives just at the end. Arrange the cooked bell peppers, olives and sun-dried tomatoes on bed of quinoa.

Black Eyed Peas with Beets and Hazelnut Salad and Pita Bread Ingredients:

115 oz. can of black-eyed peas rinsed

1 C. cooked shredded beets (canned or fresh) 1/2 C. chopped hazelnuts

Dressing: 1/4 C. balsamic vinegar 1/2 C. extra virgin olive oil

1 tsp. thyme

Rinse the black-eyed peas. Place in individual bowls. Top with beets, chopped hazelnuts and dressing.

Selves 2.

DINNER: Walnut Encrusted Salmon Ingredients:

1 lb. salmon cut in half 1/4 C. breadcrumbs 1/4 C. walnuts

1T. dijon mustard

1/2 tsp. cayenne pepper 2 T. honey

Preheat oven to 375 degrees F.

Grind walnuts in small food processor. Mix well with honey, mustard, and cayenne pepper and spread onto salmon. Bake at 375 degrees F for 20 minutes.

Serves 2. Roast Chicken with Turmeric Ingredients:

Ingredients:

4 lb. whole chicken 1 head garlic

1/4 C. extra virgin olive oil 2 tsp. sea salt

2 tsp. turmeric

1 tsp. black pepper

Preheat oven to 375 degrees F.

Rinse and dry chicken and place in roasting pan. Rub the chicken with olive oil. Mix the salt, turmeric, and black pepper together and sprinkle this over the top of the chicken, and rub some in the cavity.

Cut the head of garlic in half crosswise. Place garlic in pan with the cut side facing down.

Roast for 1 hour and check for doneness. If the flesh is pink near the bone, it will require more time. It can be covered while roasting to prevent drying out and burning the skin. It should be golden brown when finished.

Selves 4 to 6.

Lentil and Chicken Soup with Sweet Potato and Spinach

Ingredients: 3 T. extra virgin olive oil

1 medium onion chopped medium onion chopped

3 cloves garlic minced 2 carrots chopped

1/2 tsp. cayenne 1 tsp. turmeric

1 tsp. cumin

1 1/2 freshly grated ginger

4 C. low sodium chicken broth 115 oz. can coconut milk

1C. lentils

3 C. shredded chicken breast

Sea salt and black pepper to taste Garnish: Sprigs of fresh cilantro

Saute onion in olive oil on low heat for 5 minutes, stirring occasionally. Then add garlic and spices, carrots and ginger continuing to saute for another 2 minutes.

Add the chicken broth, and lentils and cook until lentils are tender. You

may need to add water to the broth.

Add coconut milk and cook until soup thickens. Taste and adjust seasoning to taste. Garnish with cilantro.

Selves 4 to 6.

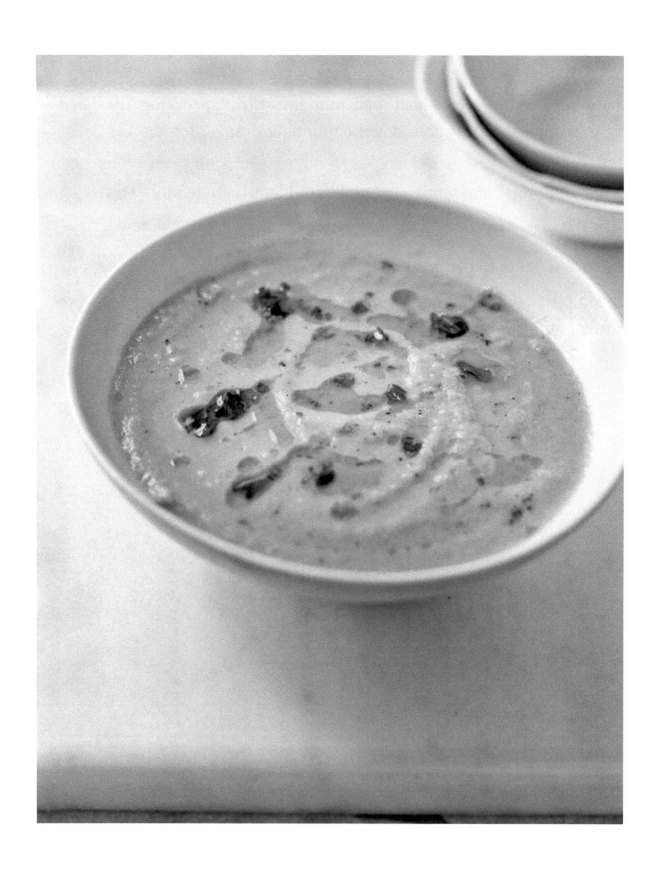

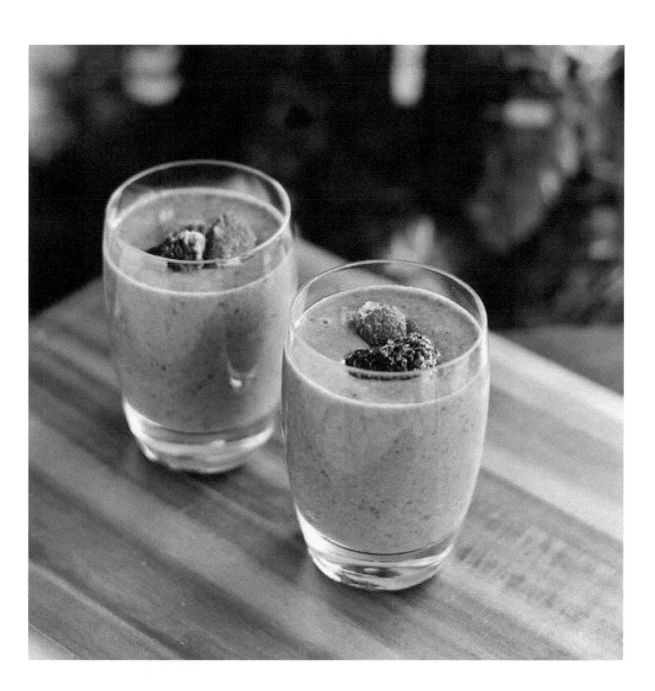

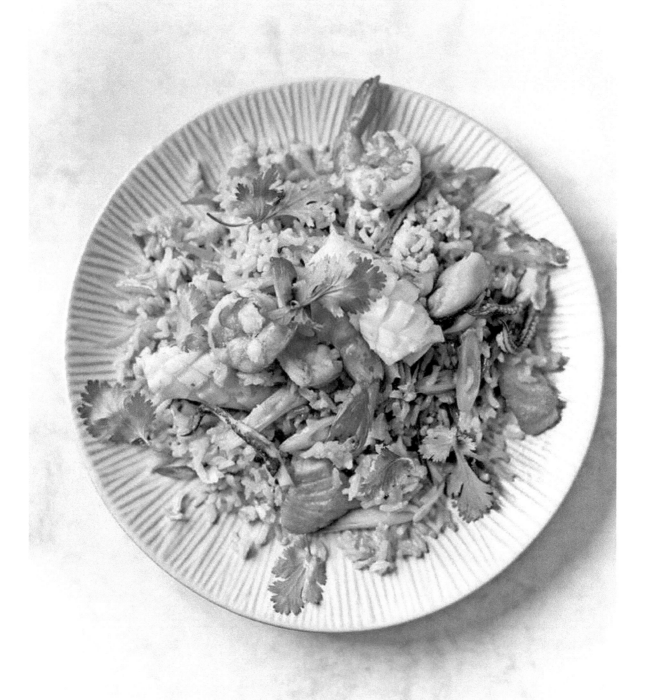

CPSIA information can be obtained
at www.ICGtesting.com
Printed in the USA
BVHW050159050122
625441BV00015B/652